# Walking Miles in Sensible Shoes

.

# Walking Miles in Sensible Shoes

## A NURSE LOOKS BACK AT HER VOCATION

*Norma Fay Nicholson*

Walking in Sensible Shoes: A Nurse Looks Back At Her Vocation

ISBN-10: 1541133307
ISBN-13: 9781541133303
Library of Congress Control Number: 2017901246
CreateSpace Independent Publishing Platform
North Charleston South Carolina

Cover by Norma Nicholson
IgnitePress
4204 Shelby Cres, Mississauga
Ontario, Canada L4W 3N5

Lived experiences of the author, all names have been changed and details of stories blurred to protect privacy.

# Contents

# Acknowledgments

*The words that enlighten the soul are
more precious than jewels.*

—Inayat Khan

Thank you, Lord, for the path you have led me into. My success today is a reflection of knowing you and all the unique and awesome people you have allowed me to interact with.

To all health-care professionals with whom I have worked, I am honored and privileged to have this experience.

To the health-care organizations that have supported my growth, like the Hospital for Sick Children, thank you for recognizing my talents.

To the clients and families with whom I have interacted and cared for through ups and downs, thank you.

To my family—especially Judith and my husband, Noel—thank you for your love and support.

To friends, nursing colleagues, and students, I owe you much for the person I am today.

Last but not the least, heartfelt thanks to Cheryl Antao-Xavier and Olive Steeles for allowing me many opportunities to pick your brains to move forward.

# CHAPTER 1

# From a Nanny to the Launching of a Nursing Career: Registered Practical Nurse

⟶

*Nothing can stop the man with the right mental attitude from achieving his goal; nothing on earth can help the man with the wrong mental attitude.*

—THOMAS JEFFERSON

"ANDREA, CLIMB DOWN FROM THAT chair please—like, now!"

Pouting, and with a frown on her face, she responded, "Norma, you hide the good cookies on the highest shelf in the cupboard. How can I get to them without climbing on the chair?"

In fact, the "good" cookies were right in front of her on the lowest shelf. She was the youngest in this household and the busy bee. She wanted cookies, and I was most concerned about her safety!

Living an exciting and blossoming life as a nanny in a household of three daughters, one son, and their parents, there was never a quiet moment except when the lights went out at nights. This home was filled with love and nurturing; you could see and feel the happiness emanating from the children. Working hard was nothing new, because I had worked to ensure my basic needs were met since the age of eight. Ensuring this family enjoyed a clean and safe environment where their children thrived was one of my major priorities, and I did this to the best of my abilities.

This family valued my positive attitude in caring for them and encouraged me to volunteer at the hospital once a week so that I could get out and see a bit more of the world. They saw my potential to move into a career when I had not even thought about moving in this direction.

"You will make a fine nurse one day, Norma," said Andrea, my youngest cheerleader in the household.

I sought out the role of a candy striper at an acute-care adult hospital. Just attending an interview to say why I wanted to be a volunteer and the skills I would bring was very gratifying. When I became a volunteer, a new world opened for me. I was in awe of how sharing words of encouragement, assisting patients to eat their meals, or just quietly sitting at their bedsides helped them not to think of their discomforts or other events that they were unable to attend to due to hospitalization.

I volunteered for one year while I continued working as a full-time nanny. Volunteering created a lasting legacy that transformed my life and the lives of the people I interacted with. It formed the base on which I built my nursing career.

Dressed in my pink-striped volunteer uniform, I began to walk more upright as a professional. I began to learn medical terminologies, what nurses needed to know, and how they applied this knowledge to care of their patients. I learned how physicians relayed information to the patients and the patients' understanding of what they were told. I was immersed in a world of health-care learning and became so engaged I obtained permission to extend the hours I volunteered to two days each week.

I saw firsthand how one person can make a difference in the lives of others. For those patients and families with whom I interacted and assisted, I may never know to the full extent how that gift of time truly impacted their lives, but I saw many smiles and received many thanks.

I daydreamed of the time when I would have the opportunity to waltz into a nursing career. Reality told me that this would not be easy, especially since I lived in someone's home where I was a nanny and did not have adequate finances to move to my own place. However, I had twelfth-grade education and the motivation to become a nurse.

As a six-month-old infant, I was abandoned on a sidewalk by my teenage mother. My paternal grandmother rescued me from the street; it was a blessing to be alive to consider a nursing career. I knew nothing came easy in life. Even with my commitment to becoming a nurse, everything wouldn't be rosy, and I might face failure in my quest to enter this profession. I thought about the times when my grandmother told me, "Little girl, you were born for a purpose. Life will test you, obstacles will arise, and you will make mistakes, but don't ever allow these challenges to prevent you from reaching your potential." My nana was so smart, and she had only a second-grade education.

With these words always at the forefront of my mind, I made an appointment with my employer to discuss my future goal of becoming a nurse. The parents and children were engaged in this discussion, and they all wanted me to succeed; nevertheless, they did not want me to leave their employment. I entered into part-time studies through the Ministry of Education to become a registered practical nurse, and I continued my full-time employment.

Classroom studies came naturally because, in my role as a volunteer, I had seen how the theories were transferred from the classroom and applied at the bedsides by practicing nurses. Excited but petrified to go into my nursing placement, I was also fearful my full-time employment would come to an end. Here was a great opportunity for me, and I wanted to take hold of it. Starting over can be scary but it can also be exciting, and with the right attitude to succeed, I said goodbye to my employer. This was done with mixed emotions on both sides. I had no family in Canada and would miss the comforts of a warm and welcoming home. I had a few close friends who assisted me with transitioning to the community, and I easily found my own apartment.

I loved to read, and I came across a quote from Ted Engstrom: "The rewards for those who persevere far exceed the pain that must precede the victory." These words gave me the courage to continue my quest to become a nurse. I was feeling awesome, and this positive attitude kept me going and enhanced my commitment to succeed.

⎯⎯⎯⎯⎯⎯⎯⎯⎯⎯⎯

### Clinical Placement as a Practical Nurse: Adult Setting

Mary Crowley said, "One person with a commitment is worth more than one hundred people who have only an interest." I had the commitment to make a difference in the lives of individuals who required health care, and I planned to succeed.

Classroom studies were held five days each week, starting at 8:00 a.m. and ending at 4:00 p.m. I adjusted to this routine very easily. Orientation to a new health-care environment was a requirement before starting a nursing placement. This was a breeze; I had been a volunteer in a hospital, so I immediately recognized the flow and processes when I entered the nursing unit. What I needed to learn quickly was the application of nursing skills to ensure individualized, respectful, and compassionate care.

I had been enjoying staying up late at night and not having to wake until 7:00 a.m. to get to classes. I was unaware of the daunting task that would be my nursing placement. Imagine having to get to bed by 8:00 p.m. so that you could be up at 5:00 a.m. Just thinking of this change made me feel tired; however, the joy of waking early to the singing birds in springtime rejuvenated me and enhanced my awareness of the accomplishments I dreamed of.

I was becoming a real nurse! When I arrived at the hospital, I headed to the locker room to change into my white starched uniform, cap, and shoes. Punctuality and flexibility were very important; the classroom teacher ensured that students understood these traits were necessary to become a good nurse. The bounce in my steps, the smile on my face, the thanks from patients and their families, and the compliments from the nurses made my day.

New patients were admitted to the hospital daily, and many were discharged home, freeing up beds for the newly admitted. What an awesome privilege it was to interact with people from different cultures and languages. I took the time to go to the library to read about cultures and to gain understanding of where health-care needs differed.

There were many opportunities to involve patients and families in their health care, ensuring timely follow-up and discharge planning were in place. I also learned quickly that it takes a team of multidisciplinary health-care professionals to assist patients' return to optimal health. I collaborated and worked with physiotherapists, occupational therapists, social workers, chaplains, other students, nurses, and a variety of physicians and community stakeholders.

I enjoyed the hustle and bustle of the nursing unit. Carts were everywhere, containing linen for bed changes and meals ready to be served. Housekeepers waited to wash the floors; porters took patients for diagnostic tests, and nurses delivered medications. The physicians visited mostly in the mornings. With the ringing of patients' bedside call bells and the telephones, I easily understood why I had the occasional headache at the end of my tour of duty.

I successfully completed my placements in two adult health-care settings without any major challenges. Great teamwork with the patient was always the center of what we did and had measurable outcomes.

I next moved to placement in Pediatrics at one of the major, renowned hospitals in the city.

GROWTH AND CHALLENGES IN PEDIATRIC PLACEMENT
When a student nurse is learning to apply classroom theories to the delivery of nursing care for infants and toddlers, it is a real change from working with adults. You look at these little ones and know you are entirely responsible for them until their parents visit and help with aspects of care. I learned more from the mistakes I made, and I became a pediatric nurse.

Having delivered nursing care to adults and engaged them in decision-making about recovery and self-care at home, I went into the pediatric setting hoping to engage parents in a like manner. The surprises and challenges came quickly. It took lots of support from a caring nursing educator and a nurse mentor to support me so that I could move forward.

When nursing care was delivered in collaboration with adult patients, one had discussions, and choices were made focusing on the health outcomes for the patients. You could provide resources and allow the patients to carry out some aspects of care (if able), such as eating their meals, managing hygiene, and getting dressed. They understood instructions or would request clarification.

Quite the opposite approach was true when delivering nursing care to infants and toddlers. Each required full care and cried often, demanding immediate attention. Could you imagine being assigned to the care of two infants and three toddlers at 7:00 a.m., where both infants were crying and the toddlers were waking up for breakfast and hugs? My nursing teacher challenged me with this assignment.

The use of Pampers or Huggies diapers was not yet acceptable in hospitals. I was taught to fold a cloth diaper in a specific manner and use large safety pins to hold this diaper in place. You had to be careful your hands were placed against the skin of the infant inside the diapers to prevent harm when the pins were inserted. Guess who got most of the pinpricks—my fingers, until I learned the correct way to do this hardy task.

I was thankful I became an integral part of a nursing team where we helped each other deliver the required care. At times, moms or dads stayed overnight with their children. I expressed daily thanks for their help in ensuring timely care for their children.

At times, I felt overwhelmed when rushing around; I was so busy striving to ensure each tiny patient was OK, as my heart skipped many beats. One morning, I went into a cubicle—an area where infants would be in cribs—to pick up an infant. I had gathered diapers, wipes, and a change of clothing for the infant. As I removed his wet diaper while he lay on his back, he peed upward into my face and all over the top of my uniform. I did not see that coming and was not prepared to prevent this mishap.

I was very flustered; I didn't know if this incident had occurred with any nurse before. I called one of my colleagues to help, changed the infant, and handed him over to her. I then changed his bedding and went to my locker room to wash my face and change my uniform. This story spread rapidly around the nursing unit. What could I do? I was embarrassed, but when teased about the little boy peeing right in my face, I had to laugh. I learned my lesson—always have an added towel when changing a boy!

I often sang to infants while sitting in a rocking chair feeding or calming them. One morning, I was engaged in this activity, and an older gentleman came to the area and asked to see an infant. I was so happy to see someone who would want to help.

"It's so nice to see a grandfather up so early to help," I said, once he identified himself as a family member and provided the name of the infant.

"This is my son. I'm not his grandfather," he responded in a terse manner.

I wished I could have hidden under the infant's crib. I apologized many times over, and I learned assumptions were not facts and should not be used. In all future contacts with parents or grandparents, I asked for their names and relation-ship with the child before getting engaged in discussions. That mistake was not repeated.

I loved working with children of all age groups, engaging families, and having the privilege of seeing great health out-comes. I experienced a few sad situations where children were handed over to the Children's Aid Society due to abuse and neglect, or some were very ill and died in the hospital.

After six weeks of Pediatrics placement, I was ready to write my provincial examination to become a practical nurse. Prior to leaving the Pediatric health-care environment, I vis-ited the human-resources department and gave my résumé to a recruiter. I was encouraged to inform the department as soon as my exam results were available.

Success! I passed my registered practical nursing exam with flying colors, and I was now prepared to work for a sal-ary doing what I loved.

## Obtained Full-Time Job as a Pediatric Registered Practical Nurse

I was invited to come to the hospital for two weeks of orien-tation. What—no interview? The recruiter told me the staff with whom I did my placement in the different Pediatric ar-eas had already delivered written references, so there was no need to have an interview.

Having completed my nursing placement in this setting, I needed to learn quickly the flow of health-care activities, and how I fit into the team dynamics. Amazingly, I enjoyed working with the patients, families, and my team. I was so engaged that, at times, I would stay several minutes past the end of my tour of duty to help a parent learn the required care their children needed.

I mastered working within a medical team, as infants, toddlers and children up to the age of ten were admitted to my medical unit. Many had type 1 diabetes, asthma, sickle cell anemia, Crohn's disease, cystic fibrosis, or cancer. This was a large unit with twenty-six children.

In the early 1970s, there was no cure for several childhood cancers and minimal treatment for sickle cell disease and cystic fibrosis. I quickly learned about approaches in palliative care to help families cope with their many losses.

One of my favorite toddlers, Chris, had lived at the hospital since birth. His lungs were plugged with the mucus produced by having cystic fibrosis. His health was too fragile for his mom to take him home. He required twenty-four-hour health care. I headed to my medical unit one afternoon at 2:45 p.m. to ensure early arrival for my evening tour of duty, to exchange information from the staff who worked the day tour.

As I stepped off the elevator and the door slowly closed, I heard a loud scream coming from Chris's room. Several nurses and a doctor were running toward the room. I stood quietly, fearing the worst. Looking down the hallway next to the nursing station, I saw the toddler's mom lying on the floor on her back and tightly holding her son.

"Somebody help!" she screamed at the top of her lungs. Chris seemed lifeless.

I was affixed to the nursing station, unable to move. There was no Code Blue—this was decided with the parents and teams—no resuscitation efforts for Chris. He died peacefully in his mother's arms.

Fast-forward to today, where new approaches in treatment have become a reality for enhancing the health of children with cystic fibrosis. I cannot help but wish there was more that could have been done to save the life of this brave toddler.

## A Bit about Cystic Fibrosis (CF)

CF is a hereditary disorder affecting the endocrine glands. This causes the production of abnormally large amounts of thick mucus, leading to the blockage of the pancreatic ducts, bronchi, intestines, kidneys, and liver. Children having this disorder experience frequent respiratory infections. The disorder is usually treated with pancreatic enzyme replacement, fat-soluble vitamins, antibiotics, and frequent chest physiotherapy.

In the 1970s, many children died at birth or by the time they were toddlers because these approaches did not always produce good results.

New developments in medicine have enormously benefited families and our society. Most children with CF now live to have families of their own. Many have accessed lung and liver transplants and are living healthy.

## The Death of My Favorite Eight-Year-Old Patient

I often wonder what it is about elevators, this form of vertical transportation that moves people or goods from floor to floor. Is it because I get on an elevator daily and travel to the eighth floor, the topmost level? Each time the elevator opens into the middle of my medical unit, someone stops what they are doing to see who comes onto our floor.

The pediatric hospital had a heliport and when a helicopter arrived, an announcement was made over the PA system. All employees knew they should stay far away for safety reasons. We also knew something serious had occurred and a child needed dire emergency treatment to have been brought to the hospital by a helicopter.

In our unit, we went about delivering care, knowing this emergency involved only staff who worked in the Emergency Department of the hospital. My manager informed us she would go to the Emergency Department to see if any additional help was needed. She took the special Emergency Department elevator to the ground level and entered the department. To her surprise, she observed one of our past patients and his dad were sitting outside the elevator, with many medical personnel telling him they could not go to the eighth floor before being seen in the Emergency Department.

This dad was adamant that he wanted no one to touch his son until they were in the medical unit. He also stated he did not want anyone to accompany them into the elevator. No one could override this decision, as this dad was very firm in what he wanted to occur. The Emergency Department team took another elevator to get them to the eighth floor.

Remember, I asked myself, what was it about elevators? The door slowly opened, and I saw James's dad holding him close to his body. What the heck was happening here? I found courage to walk to the elevator and took James in my arms. His dad fainted to the side of the opened elevator, and other nurses hurriedly took care of him. With James in my arms, I walked briskly to the nearest treatment room. Ensuring that no one was on the stretcher, I laid James on the stretcher.

I am sharing this story with you, my readers, and I must stop for a few minutes, because emotionally I am in that moment in the treatment room, when all the doctors and nurses walked in and found that James had died. I became weak, and I too must have fainted. The next thing I remember is that I was awake, sitting in a chair in my manager's office.

James had leukemia and was discharged from our unit two weeks previously because there was no further treatment to help him get well. He had spent six months in our unit, and his dad was accommodated to spend as much time as he could with his son. His wife and the other children were at home (Unable to fix here!).

As his health deteriorated, his parents wanted to take him home to provide palliative care with the help of community nurses. They were very rich; they owned the helicopter that brought James to the hospital. When they left home north of the city, they sensed he was dying because of the signs and symptoms he demonstrated. In their moment of despair, the only place they now wanted him to die was with the nurse who spent hours with James, even on her day off. For as long as I have been a nurse, that moment has been sealed in my mind.

That was a great life-altering experience for me. Until that day, I had not held a child or person who had died. I had no doubt my career in nursing was worth all the effort I had put into it, but I wondered if I had the stamina to participate in such grief. As a nurse of over forty years, I have assisted families many times in managing the death of children and adults.

There were many happy situations where very ill children came to the hospital, and our team thought they would not be well again. Surprisingly, they went home with their parents, returning to full and healthy lives. This is the part that kept me loving what I do. Our team always celebrated those happy occasions.

# CHAPTER 2

# On Becoming a Registered Nurse

⤜

*The rewards for those who persevere far exceed
the pain that must precede the victory.*

—TED ENGSTROM

WORKING AS A REGISTERED PRACTICAL nurse gave me great insights into life and death. A patient could be alive and talking with me about wanting to go home, and in one minute, that patient may go into cardiac arrest. The patient might die within two minutes. This would be expected by the healthcare team and family, so no surprise. However, I was reminded every day that life is a gift and it is up to me to learn to receive it, because this gift could be lost in one breath.

I worked in a caring environment, in which collaboration and partnering were the norm. We helped each other in the delivery of health care to a vast variety of patients, and I became more mature, more organized, and highly educated.

There were times I wished that I could become a registered nurse. I had gained so many skills over eight years as an RPN that I was assigned to facilitate orientation for newly hired RNs to my unit. I had the skills to do more, but was prohibited by my role and registration status.

My circumstances changed as I worked through an evening tour of duty. In the medical unit, there were twenty-six patients, between eighteen months and eight years of age. Two registered nurses and two registered practical nurses were on duty. The duty assignments were completed by the manager of the unit according to the acuity of the patients. I worked with an RN that evening to deliver care to ten of the youngest patients, all with IVs in their arms or legs. I needed roller blades, but running shoes had to get me around.

The registered nurses organized their work to ensure all patients received the best care possible. In the evenings, the focus remained mostly on assessments, nutrition, timely monitoring, and delivery of medication. To facilitate easy access to intravenous fluids for each patient, the RNs prepared the bags of clearly labeled medication and locked them in cupboards above each patient's bed or crib.

I went in a room to visit an infant who had an IV inserted in her arm. I assessed the infant, checked the site, the flow rate of the fluid, and the remaining amount of fluid in the medication bag. I did all this, and noticed the medication bag was empty and the tubing attached to the infant's arm would be empty soon if a new medication bag was not hung as soon as possible. Knowing the RN was in another room trying to restart an IV on a toddler—and the medication was above the crib—I took it from the cupboard, checked the name against the infant's arm bracelet, removed the empty bag, and hung the new one. I was so focused on ensuring everything was safe and so happy the IV site was kept patent that I did not hear the footsteps of the supervisor coming into the room.

I felt a tap on my right shoulder and spun around to see the supervisor glaring at me. I did not know what to say, because this was not a part of my duty.

She spoke first. "What do you think you're doing? This isn't the role of a registered practical nurse."

I explained I did not want the infant, who was so ill and had very few veins, to have a blocked intravenous site. I also informed her I had done all the necessary checks to ensure safety, and I was on my way to inform the RN about what I had done so that she could recheck and document the change of fluids.

The supervisor thanked me for smart thinking. She also requested that, before I came on duty the following day, I stop by the Nursing Administration Department for further discussion. I knew at times we could control our circumstances, but at that moment, I felt I could control neither my circumstances nor my thoughts. I began to think the worst; to me, that meant I would have no job in twenty-four hours. I completed my tour of duty safely and was humbled I had acquired the skills to help an infant in this way. The RN expressed gratitude for my action.

My negative thoughts continued on my way home, and I found it impossible to sleep. What if I went to the administration the next day and was told I was fired because of what I had done? I was awake by 7:00 a.m. with a headache. I called the unit to speak with my manager, but she was too busy to have a discussion. I felt alone and unable to focus on any task at home, except watching TV. I went to work a half hour before it was time to go on duty. With much hesitation, I entered the administrative office and asked to see the evening supervisor.

She welcomed me into her office, and then I saw the vice president of nursing and my manager walking to the office. I was sure this was the moment of my demise. I had the opportunity to be seated, but stood instead. I eagerly wanted to know the reason for the meeting. I felt that if I was standing, it would be easier to walk out of the office.

My manager spoke first and informed me she received wonderful feedback from the supervisor about my work ethic. I felt my heart slow, and my headache diminish. I asked what she was told, but instead of responding, she asked, "Do you want to become a registered nurse?"

I did not believe what I was hearing. Instead of saying yes, I responded that such a goal was not achievable for me due to finances. The supervisor told me this was not the first time she had heard about my work ethic and, having seen my dedication herself, she recommended to the vice president that the hospital support me with an education fund to obtain my RN.

There were no words to express my happiness on hearing such an offer. Lots of happy tears flowed. I accepted gracefully and signed a contract, which requested that, after graduation and successful completion of my provincial examination, I return to work in the capacity of a registered nurse for a minimum of three years. Who could ever say no to such an offer? Another dream was coming through for me as a whole new world opened with greater opportunities.

Many blessings came my way: I was accepted and enrolled into the nursing diploma program at George Brown College, and my tuition and books were paid for by the hospital. I had access to the medical library to aid my studies, networked with many colleagues who mentored me through the three years of study, and received an Ontario grant to pay other bills. What more could a person ask for, except to give thanks and ensure successful completion of my studies.

### Placement as an RN Student

I completed my entire required placements at the hospital where I volunteered and at the children's hospital where I was employed as an RPN.

Life was never without challenges, and one could become despondent in response to those situations, but negative responses do not build character. I often listened to another perspective and, where possible, responded in a calm manner.

In the adult setting, I was assigned to a patient who was seven days postoperative. She was a diabetic and had a left below-knee amputation. Her plans of care directed me to support her continued participation in her rehabilitation by demonstrating how she was able to change her bandage daily and ambulate from bed to chair. The patient and I agreed I would observe how she did her bandaging after morning care and breakfast. The patient followed through and did all tasks efficiently while I stood by and observed, prepared to assist when required. She then went in her wheelchair to the recreation area.

My nursing educator came to the unit to assess how I managed the care for this patient. I took the plan of care and explained how the tasks were carried out. She directed me to get the patient back to bed, as she needed to observe me changing the bandage. She stated I was a student and must be observed completing new tasks. I explained I was unaware she wanted to observe, and I would let her do so the following morning. She insisted I go to the recreation area and return the patient to her room. Deep breaths helped, and I took many before I was able to respond to this request from the educator.

I asked the educator to accompany me to see the patient in that setting, because I could not return the patient if she was already engaged in an activity. I was sure an angel followed me along the hallway—the patient was engaged in a recreational activity, did not want to leave, and suggested the educator trust her student would do a great job.

Later that day, I respectfully spoke with my nursing educator and informed her I had been a registered practical nurse for eight years, and had changed many bandages during that time. I was relieved she did not challenge me about other nursing tasks. She asked me to become a mentor for the other four nursing students in the unit. I gladly accepted that role.

I kept in touch with my multidisciplinary colleagues and worked casually with them while attending college. After successful completion of my studies, my placements, and my provincial exam, I returned to a full-time registered nursing role in the hospital. I was accepted to the unit where I had previously worked as an RPN.

## On Becoming a Gainfully Employed RN

Initially, I thought it was great. I could return to my old work area, where my growth was nurtured; however, I found out quickly this was not the best choice. Over the three years I attended college, the twenty-six-bed unit was now assigned to two groups of patients, most of whom had type 1 diabetes.

The morning routine for the patients with diabetes was to have all those who were able to administer their insulin gather in the large treatment room. Each patient completed blood sugar checks and then prepared their insulin. A registered nurse is required to check each patient's medical order for insulin and ensure the patient draws the correct amount of insulin from a vial and injects by the subcutaneous route.

There are now insulin pens that are much easier to manage, even by a four-year-old child.

I offered to work with the patients that morning. There were ten patients who required this support, and after I assisted seven, the charge nurse came into the treatment room.

"Norma, what do you think you're doing?" she asked loudly.

"Assisting these guys with their morning routines so that they can go have their breakfast," I responded.

She asked me to leave the room and stated she would complete the tasks. I exited and went to the manager's office. I was very upset about the situation that had occurred and had been carried out in front of the patients. I asked my manager to facilitate a transfer to another area when there was a vacancy. I did not like what had occurred. I became afraid that a similar situation would occur again.

When all the patients completed their prebreakfast routines and went to the dining room, I asked to speak with the charge nurse. She apologized several times over and stated she had previously seen me in the role of an RPN, where I was not allowed to monitor patients who have diabetes. In that moment, she did not remember I was now an RN and had the ability and right to carry out such tasks. I suggested she could have had a private discussion away from the patients and not embarrass me in such a manner.

I forgave her, as we are all prone to see actions from our past being used to guide our present activities. We all make mistakes, and sometimes there was no way to go back and fix it, but we could move forward wiser and in control of our lives.

I now realize this was a form of bullying in the workplace.

I decided I still wanted to be transferred where I would meet new colleagues. My manager completed the transfer form, and I knew this would take time to occur until there was a vacancy in another unit for the skills of an RN.

It took a while to build trust with the patients in my unit. They asked about my role and how safe it was to have me on the unit. Parents were invited to attend a short meeting along with their children. Discussion occurred so that all of them understood I was qualified to do the work, and the charge nurse apologized to everyone for her actions.

It was so good to have a mentor who was a great friend. It made the rough spots in life less difficult. After this incident, I had an opportunity to meet with my mentor, a wonderful physician who remained a friend forty years later. She taught me how to become assertive, to communicate my ideas, preferences, and feelings in a clear and direct manner. She assisted me in understanding that assertiveness was especially crucial during times of transition, because what I was used to doing and having presently in my life had changed. The connections and contacts I needed from nursing colleagues were different from what had worked before the transition. In being assertive, I had to believe it was worth having others displeased momentarily with me in order to get what was important to me.

Dare to be different! I grew into a dynamic nursing leader. A new start in a different area brought much learning. I reminded myself it did not matter where I came from, what I had been through, or my social-economic status; what really mattered was the love and passion I had as a registered nurse.

Ann Landers said, "Opportunities are usually disguised as hard work, so most people don't recognize them." My mentor assisted me in becoming aware of many opportunities. Within two years of becoming an RN, I followed up on a job posting and was accepted to be one of the hospital's educators. I continued to do small things with great love.

I became a mentor and coach with the ability to practice my most important values and beliefs. In my new work area, it was ensuring a warm work environment where every member of the team felt valued. I also coached the nurses in realizing their strengths and how to build on them so that they could be an integral part of their team, while serving the patients and families beyond their expectations.

I served at this children's hospital for sixteen years, with an equal number of years in the roles of RPN and RN. I have many great memories from this experience: I was given opportunities to thrive and grow, and I accepted each challenge with grace and honor. Most of our lives are spent in the midst of change; I accepted my next opportunity and moved to an adult acute-care hospital to become a nurse manager.

## Much Ongoing Learning

*Don't fear alone-time.*
*Don't dwell on the past.*
*Don't feel the world owes you.*
*Don't expect immediate results.*
*Don't worry about pleasing everyone.*
*Don't waste time feeling sorry for yourself.*
*Don't waste energy on things you can't control.*
*Don't let others influence your emotions.*
*Don't resent other people's success.*
*Don't shy away from responsibility.*
*Don't give up after first failure.*
*Don't fear taking calculated risks.*

(Adsense 987052)

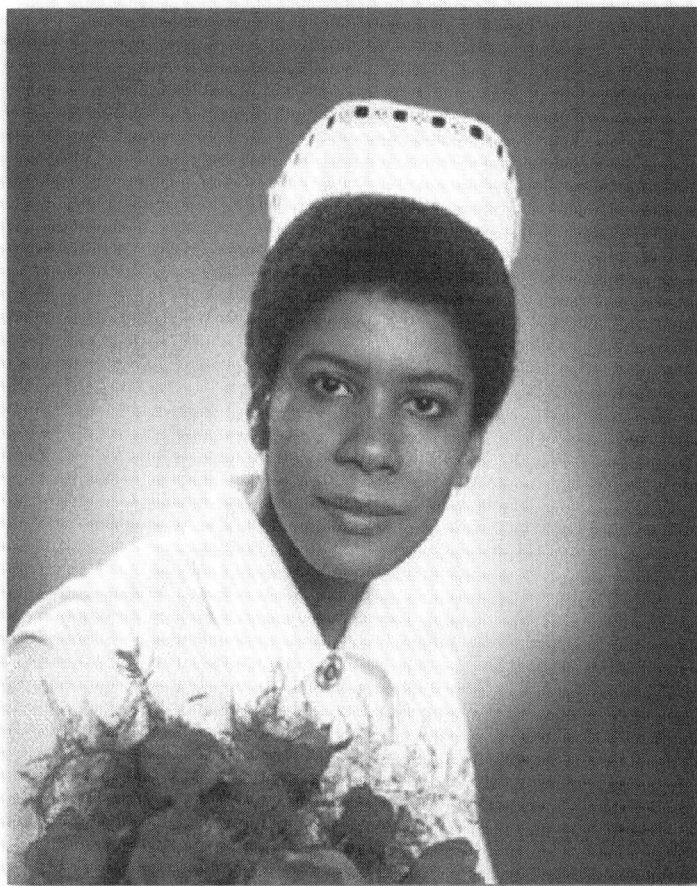

RN Graduate, George Brown College

# CHAPTER 3

# Entering a Leadership Role as a Nurse Manager

﹏

*When you see something beautiful in someone,*
*tell that person. It may take seconds for you to say,*
*but for that person, this may last a lifetime.*

—*Unknown*

I HAPPILY ATTENDED AN INTERVIEW and accepted a new job in an adult acute hospital in a surgical unit.

"Norma, you can do this," my mentor said.

My first day on the job, I was filled with pride and excitement mixed with anxiety. I was taking on a new role and unsure how it would play out. But I reminded myself that taking risks and learning were part of becoming more mature.

I now had two mentors who met with me separately each week over lunch or coffee. I had been nurtured to know there was no such thing as overnight success. In fact, my goal was to become successful, not necessarily a success. When you focus on success, you often measure your progress by the world's standards. I did not want to compete with others to see if I had the right home, car, clothes, club membership, and so on—just like the Joneses. My goal was to do the very best I could in whatever I do and to give back to society.

I revisited my values and realized they had developed even further. I also learned one of the secrets to personal fulfillment and career success was being able to integrate my values, beliefs, and purpose into everything I did, including work. I wanted my work and career to be an extension of who I was and to provide me with opportunities for personal fulfillment.

## My Values Revisited

**Gratitude:** I awaken each morning with a sense of gratitude and retire at night with a sense of gratitude. I am so thankful to be alive and for the opportunities I have as a Canadian citizen. I love the Lord, my family, good friends, and my church. I have opportunities to improve my life each day, and I give back freely to society, not expecting anything in return.

**Family:** I could not survive without my family. They are an integral part of my being. I am fed by their love, and in return, I am so blessed. My family is not only those connected to me by heredity, but also those who helped me realize my dreams.

**Growth:** I am a lifelong learner, which creates wonderful opportunities for me to have visions and to move into the future. New learning gives me a zest for life, as I am always inquisitive. I get excited when an opportunity for me to learn is presented.

**Honesty:** I enjoy the company of folks who are honest. I dislike gossip and tend to walk away from such conversations. I would rather talk to someone than gossip behind his or her back. My friendships are built on honesty.

**Freedom:** This helps me to make decisions to work where I want, develop my skills, have unique friends, and make good choices. I live in a country of my choice, where there are no restrictions on my religion as a Christian. I love the freedom to be informed, to be able to bring diverse perspectives together, and to stay focused.


Surgical Inpatient Setting: Adult Hospital

I was a new nurse manager; a newbie on the block; and excited to attend orientation, which included training in health-care leadership and management. As I read my job description and clarified some of the responsibilities, I became more aware of the enormous responsibilities I had undertaken.

Having worked as a health-care educator, I enjoyed my interactions with the staff and the patients. There were days when being an educator was really fun. Nurses would be supported to learn about starting an IV or carrying out a post-operative assessment. They would later forget some of the instructions.

"Norma, how is it you don't get upset when we forget the instructions you taught us?" they asked.

"That's why you now have the opportunity to demonstrate the techniques on a mannequin before getting to the patients," I responded.

In this new role of manager, I knew having a positive attitude and collaborating with our interdisciplinary team would ensure excellence in nursing care, as well as ongoing education for them to be the best health-care practitioners they could. I now had the opportunity to learn systems approach in health care, and I was happy for the opportunity to assist the staff's growth even more.

Remember my two mentors? I needed to spend more time with them to gain new ideas and quickly learn additional skills to collaborate and build our health-care team, and partner with the doctors, senior management, and our community—building schedules, monitoring the budget, attending management meetings—what had I gotten myself into?

I met my new team, and many were still grieving from the departure of their past manager. This individual had retired, and the staff verbalized their fear that everything would change in their work area. I confirmed I was indeed different, and changes would occur, but not without their input. I was committed to learning about all staff members and what their goals were by scheduling one-to-one and small-group meetings. I also connected with the physicians one-to-one and on service levels.

Our first staff meeting was called "getting to know." I shared that each of us needed to develop goals, always be on the lookout to add value to the care we brought our patients, and engage the patients in planning and carrying out their health care. I also informed my team I needed to know about the good things they were doing and areas that presented challenges. Along with informing me about challenges, I looked to them to suggest solutions. I was committed to working with them to develop ways in which we could collaborate with everyone, including our patients, so that we could measure outcomes and make changes.

I challenged them with the following questions, and I encouraged them to discuss and share, and together we would develop solutions:

* How will I know when I am doing well?
* What do I need to learn to do my best?
* Who do I need to help me?
* Where do I start?

Staff meetings were great ways to give each person an opportunity to bring a diverse perspective together and stay focused. This was where good-change planning could happen, as folks felt informed and engaged. We scheduled monthly staff meetings, and I ensured we had shift rotation, staff input in the agenda, and documented minutes for those who were unable to attend. We agreed on having one meeting each month, unless there was an emergency situation requiring immediate attention.

Within six months of being a manager, I got to know the staff, physicians, and other team members fairly well. I was ready to suggest a few changes but focus on one change at a time. I needed buy-in from the team for success. On the staff meeting agenda, I added an item for patient education. I observed that patients who were capable of assisting with self-care were often waiting on the nurses to complete these aspects of care. Waiting sometimes impacted on the patient's need for early ambulation from one of the rehabilitation staff.

On my walk around the unit each morning, and in having one-to-one discussions with patients, I learned nurses were always busy and preferred to do the tasks, rather than allow the patients to try, fail, and perhaps succeed the next time. I encouraged patients to share their ideas and also reminded them that changes take time. I would ensure input from others involved with their care. I made no judgment on what was occurring, but I would look at ways in which we could all engage the patients in their self-care.

## Suggestions from Patients

- Hire more staff.
- Facilitate small group discussions for patients with similar health needs.
- Add a white board to the wall in each patient's room and note how a patient could help with self-care.
- Ensure resources are easily accessible.
- Ensure safety, education, practice, and observation before increasing their involvement in self-care.

- Ensure their doctors and families know about this new approach.
- Provide educational channels on the TVs in the lounge.

As a nurse, I was always teaching and supporting patients and families. I was quite aware that when someone else's idea was not foisted upon folks, and they had some say in what they were learning, there were good outcomes. Patients engaged well when you build on what they already knew, and so do nurses.

Constant change was our reality in the world and involving folks who will be affected was a proven way to do this. I was willing to facilitate change for the improvement of health care for our patients.

I met one-on-one with random members of the multidisciplinary team to obtain information on potential solutions to ensure different approaches for patient education. We spoke over a morning coffee when allowed. I asked each person to bring suggestions to the meeting so we could develop a list of possible ways to help our patients become more independent. The next step would be to prioritize what could be done in the short term, and what needed a longer time to plan for action. We also discussed budgetary implications, as these would need to be approved by the nursing administration.

A wonderful staff meeting, or so I thought, with many suggestions aligned to those from the patients and staff. Two staff nurses verbalized fear of any change as this was perceived as patients running the ward, and the nurses would no longer be in charge. I agreed to meet with each nurse to assist in understanding the urgency and the kind of support they would receive.

We agreed that a small working group would develop a draft plan. The small group included nurses, physicians, a physiotherapist, an occupational therapist, a pharmacist, and our one and only social worker. They planned four short meetings to arrive at a draft plan. I supported this move by allocating space and time to attend, providing snacks, and being available for questions or clarification.

**The task at hand**: How do we support, educate, and engage our patients in self-care postoperatively and incorporate discharge planning to shorten their length of stay in hospital? The working group collaborated with colleagues, suggested the following, and posted this information on a white board inside the nurses' report room. They were available for all to review, to clarify, and suggest changes before a work plan was developed.

Draft Plan: Safety as a Priority

*   When the registered nurse and physician make patient rounds early each morning, include other members of the interdisciplinary team, such as a physiotherapist, occupational therapist, dietitian, discharge planner, or social worker.

- The rehabilitation staff would assess the patients, ambulate them, discuss safety, and then update their plans of care regarding their capabilities.
- The charge nurse and the patient-care assigned nurses would follow the plans of care and teach the patients aspects of self-care identified as safe for each to carry out. Opportunities would be built in for the team to clarify and change as required.
- Inform and engage all team members, including the pharmacist and the chaplain.
- The charge nurse would initiate a pilot project with a small group of patients in one wing of the unit.
- We would then evaluate outcomes and make required changes before engaging all patients in the unit.

A physician supported us in presenting our plan to our senior administration. They supported us in moving ahead. Though this meant additional work for me, I volunteered to complete the weekly evaluations with the patients and collaborate with the charge nurse to make changes to their plans of care as required.

Changes occurred every day in our lives, and at times we needed help in managing change successfully. The success or failure of this venture was dependent on the group to make decisions. No matter how good the team was, they would make mistakes and have to take corrective actions.

These two nurses wanted nothing to do with increasing the engagement of their patients. They were major complainers and were quite disgruntled, though I spent additional time communicating with them, listening to their concerns, and working out solutions together. Nothing was right for them. Even trying to encourage them to be champions of the change had no impact on their negative behavior. It was time for an individual meeting with each nurse to hear their stories and find out what additional support they required in understanding patient-centered care and the ways I would like to see them engaging in.

In separate meetings, each nurse expressed fear in using different approaches contrary to what they had used for over fifteen years. I listened, validated their concerns, and invited them to communicate specific needs. I also assisted them in understanding the major changes for the future of health care. I expressed the urgency for changes and reiterated we could not be complacent.

One nurse was adamant that she wanted nothing to do with our goals and requested a transfer from the surgical unit. The other nurse, with ongoing support, identified the skills she required to be an effective member of the team. Proud of her openness in communicating her needs as best as she could, she slowly became an integral part of the change.

Much had to be done over one year in working with the staff to effect changes. We strived to work together as a team, with open communication and engagement of patients. We encouraged each other, and over time, I observed that we had increased the number of champions for this change. There were recognition structures put in place, such as engaging the team in nominating a member who was providing outstanding support for a team member or a patient. We developed short presentations for other staff on surgical units in the hospital, and got more buy-in from the senior administration. I assisted the team in making the connections between new ways of patient care and the success of our hospital.

Have you ever been a leader or manager of a project where you have taken home all the burden each day? I constantly thought about what we could do to ensure success, and if we failed, what strategies would we use to get us back on track? We had good intentions and enthusiasm, but had to work hard to mobilize our group, as well as planning, managing change, and evaluating outcomes.

Trying to keep up with supporting the staff daily through changes, I thought about the role of an educator in supporting ongoing education to move the staff in the process of change. I developed a draft proposal to ask for an educator our unit could share with the outpatient surgical team. I met with the manager for that area to discuss this proposal, and asked her support in moving this forward. She readily supported me, as this was also one of her visions for her department. As colleagues, we had several meetings on changes in health-care approaches and what we could do to manage proactively.

The human-resources personnel assisted us in developing a tried and true proposal, with all risks identified as well as ways to manage them.

Kudos to our team—we got approval for the hiring of an educator, and both units' budgets were increased for salaries and benefits.

In the Midst of Change, Sometimes There Is Distraction

On one of my weekends at home, I planned some quiet time with my family and to use some downtime to study. I was a part-time student at the University of Toronto, and my goal was the completion of a bachelor's degree.

I received a phone call early on a Sunday morning, with a request that I come to the hospital. I asked what the emergency was, and I was told by my director we were meeting with our health-care team to look at a serious situation that had occurred in my nursing unit.

A policy in place stated a community hospital would not accept acute-care patient transfers on the weekend since there were only on-call physicians and a nurse manager to oversee anything untoward. All hospitals were staffed with decreased numbers of personnel on the weekends due to low patient-activity levels. (Except the Emergency Department, which maintained the same number of staff for all tours of duty every day.)

On my arrival at the hospital, I was informed a patient was accepted by the on-call physician from a downtown acute-care setting because that hospital was overwhelmed with patients requiring intensive-care beds in their Emergency Department. This patient was acutely ill and required one-to-one nursing care. The manager on call worked with my unit's staff to call in off-duty nurses able to work overtime tours.

Once staffing was increased to provide care to the patient, the transfer occurred. On a surgical orthopedic unit, there are not many opportunities for the staff to use their skills in the suctioning of patients. This is one of many nursing skills where the nurses are recertified annually; in that time, some may not have carried out this skill on a patient.

My understanding is that nurses did their best to ensure good health care for this patient, but he died during their tour of duty. The coroner was engaged as the patient died within twenty-four hours of being admitted. The inquest outcome noted that effective suctioning was not done to keep the patient's airway patent.

A few elderly patients had previously died in our unit, and we saw the changes and decline in those patients prior to their deaths. Physicians, patients, and families were engaged in planning whether those patients would die in the hospital setting, go to palliative care, or return home where they would die with community engagement. There was no previous example of a patient who died within a few hours of being admitted.

Other recommendations from the coroner were for increased staffing and retraining of staff. The long-term plan was policy alignment with other acute-care hospitals and partnerships.

I attended the five days of the coroner's inquest. My director blamed me for the death of the patient. She said I should have taken the time to have nurses practice this skill more frequently. What she said made no sense to me, and I felt deeply troubled. She did not provide any coverage for my unit while I was away, and this had a very negative impact on the staff, especially the nurses. At the end of each day I attended the inquest, I stopped in to check on my staff and to listen to any issues or concerns.

My vice president accompanied me to the inquest every day, and asked why I did not allow her to drop me at my home. I apprised her of what was happening in the nursing unit. She spoke with my director, and advised her to provide coverage and also to have small group discussions with the nurses with the help of the chaplain and an outside counselor. Many of the staff were traumatized by this event, especially those who worked that weekend.

Over time, and after many sessions of counseling, the team came back together. Sadly, the nurse who was assigned to the patient left her nursing career. I too sought counseling with an outside agency, as I found it very difficult to interact with my director any longer. Each time I was invited to her office regarding budgets or any other managerial concerns, she would talk about this patient.

Reflecting on that past situation, I was not brave enough to suggest that she herself needed a bit of counseling so that she could move on with her life. She strived to make my work life a *living hell*. When it was time to develop the annual budget for staffing and resources for patient care, there was a routine whereby all managers completed the first draft from the template given by the payroll department. I collaborated with other managers, and we completed these templates in a timely manner.

I made an appointment to meet with my director to review the document. She granted me time late in the evening, when I would have been at home. I brought my supper, ate at 5:00 p.m., and then went to the 6:00 p.m. meeting with her. After looking over my detailed budget template, she suggested I use a new one she had developed for surgical services, which was not yet approved by the payroll department.

As I recall this situation now, I can still feel my heart rate increasing. I do not know where I got the guts to respond.

"We need to meet with the vice president, as I will no longer take your abuses," I said.

I left her office, took my document, and went home. The following day, I scheduled a meeting with the vice president and requested a transfer to another director. After a meeting was held with all parties, my request was granted.

One hundred years from now, it will not matter that there was a disagreement with my boss. What mattered most was that I was able to stand up for myself. I remain proud of that moment, when I decided being treated in a disrespectful manner was not what I wanted for myself. I worked well with the new director until she retired. No matter how hard I tried, I was more cautious than ever due to the experience with my past director. I began to doubt whether my skills as a leader were effective as a change agent. I also had to provide added support to my staff as we continued to change protocols in our unit.

Several times, my mentors advised me that the only way to grow or learn was by experiencing my own mistakes and achievements. This was difficult; I did not make any mistakes even when I reflect on what could have been done differently.

However, I strived to push past this negative situation to find a direction.

I did not realize that there was still some anger in me about the way I was treated after the death of the patient. My ex-director became very ill with a respiratory disease. She could no longer work and was admitted to a rehab facility. During her stay, many managers and physicians visited her. She would occasionally send messages saying she would like me to visit her, and I did not respond.

On her death bed, I am told, while she was gasping for air, she asked a visitor to write a note stating she was sorry for the way she treated me. When I received this note—now I am ashamed of my response, but not then; heck, that was my best—my response to the messenger was, "Tell her to burn in hell, because she made my nursing life hell on earth." She died; I did not attend the funeral and would not know if she is in heaven or hell, and I don't care.

It was very cathartic to be able to do this. However, on reflection, this response did not reflect my value as a nurse. I now think that bad things happen and people are not perfect. I had a right to feel angry, but I did not have the right to hold on to that or feed it with more fuel. The situation was now over, I had survived, and I had moved on.

Even when stressful situations occurred in hospital settings, one or two patients always made my day by sharing information about themselves.

After I arrived in my office on a Monday morning, the charge nurse of the unit requested I join the day team during their morning report. The team wanted tips on how to effectively deliver care to an elderly male patient they viewed as having challenging behavior.

Their Story

Mr. G was an *old* man who had right-knee surgery and had been with us for the past two days while he was recovering. He ambulated with help during the day and was able to use the bathroom to void. At night, to ensure safety, he was given a urinal. I asked the male nurse to show him how to lie on his side when using the urinal. We did not know what to do, because Mr. G refused to use the urinal at night and peed in the coffee cup.

"This is so disgusting. Only you can talk with him!" the team said.

I asked if two nurses could assist the patient to the bathroom at night. They responded that they would also require the help of a physiotherapist. I agreed to help by going to visit the patient.

I went to the patient's room and knocked on the partially closed door, and he answered, "Come in." I introduced myself, and asked if it was a good time to have a short conversation over the challenges he had in the night. I also told him how sorry I was to hear he was having such a difficult time. He asked me to close the door so that no one would hear his response. He explained that all the nurses are "young girls and boys," and he did not feel comfortable telling them why it was so difficult to use a urinal.

He said, "Manager, thank you for coming to see me. I have a very short penis; it's like a short stump, and it was used to sire five children with my wife. As I get older, it seems to shrink and can't go past the top of the urinal. It's not long enough to pee into the urinal. That's why I need to use the coffee mug. The nurses are upset, but none seem to care or have asked why. Each kept asking, 'Why are you not using the urinal? What you're doing is wrong!' I hope you can solve this problem so that the nurses don't continue to be mad at me and also to talk with their colleagues about my problems."

I thanked him for sharing his concerns and promised I would discuss an alternative he could use. There was a light plastic bedpan with a small and curved top, and this would make it easier to pee into than a urinal. Should there be any other challenges he faced while hospitalized, I told him I would work with the nurses to ensure we helped him to resolve it in a shorter time.

There were four nurses on duty and a charge nurse. I asked all to come to the office, though there was only one assigned to Mr. G's care. At any time, one of these nurses could be asked to assist with the care of a patient to which he or she was not assigned. Each muffled their laughter when I told them why the patient used an alternative to the urinal.

Each nurse was asked to share examples of how each would ensure the patient received respectful and compassionate care in the future. I also thanked them for bringing this challenge to my attention so that together we could deliver the best care to all our patients.

The explanation the patient gave was as surprising to me as the nurses. I first thought he might have been experiencing pain when he tried to turn on his side by himself to use the urinal. I did not think that his challenge was related to the length of his penis.

Stranger things have happened in hospitals, and so we encouraged each other to talk with the patient and really listen. Sometimes nonverbal cues shown by the patient were good indicators to initiate conversations.

## On Becoming an Educator for Staff and Patients

What happened to my role as a manager? I wanted to respond to negativity by helping with a positive solution. I decided to become an educator. I had a sincere desire to make a difference in how nursing staff learned, and I was unable to invest much attention to that aspect of nursing in the role of a manager. The focus of leading a team into changes and the delivery of results were enormously important and time-consuming.

Some of the dollars for inpatient health care were now being transferred to outpatients and community care.

I had seen firsthand how difficult it was for my team to learn quickly about change, implementation, and measuring outcomes. I collaborated with non-health-care professionals to develop a proposal for the role of an educator for an inpatient and outpatient setting. Innovative spirit, to develop my own job description…

I was worried about what my colleagues and director would think, but I went ahead and presented the proposal to the senior team.

I think of all the time I spent worrying about what others were thinking, and to my surprise, they were thinking of their own lives most of the time. A manager colleague asked if I could tell her more about my role in the surgical unit. She would later transfer into that role, knowing she would have an excellent educator to help her staff.

Human-resources personnel developed the job description and payroll budgeted for the addition of an educator for surgery.

I was brave—having a bachelor's degree was a requirement to access this job opportunity. I applied for this position before I graduated with my degree. I had to sign on the dotted line that I would complete my degree so that a copy of the document could be added to my files. This motivated me to obtain my degree as soon as I could.

I began to spend lots of time thinking and planning how to teach, to achieve my goal. Venus Williams said, "You have to believe in yourself when no one else does. That's what makes you a winner."

I began a new career path in nursing. I believed in myself and developed into a great educator. In addition to teaching nurses, patients, and families, I began teaching in the nursing program at Sheridan College on a casual basis. My college focus was mental illness in adults and managing challenging behavior in children.

I brought back life to my career, and I could not have done so without my mentors and believing in myself, that I can change and adapt to new situations. I was much happier in an educator's role than as a manager in an acute-care setting.

Dr. Martin Luther King Jr. said, "Darkness cannot drive out darkness; only light can. Hate cannot drive out hate; only love can." I hold these words dearly. The magic that started to seep into my life when I learned to love what I was doing again was incomprehensible. My life was on an upswing when I began to truly believe in myself and the skills I had achieved.

Mergers and Stuff

Mergers of hospitals in Ontario increased rapidly in the 1990s. With much planning at all levels of provincial government and hospital administration, my hospital was converted to an urgent-care center. All inpatients were moved to the larger partner hospital. There was one CEO, one board, and a decrease in the number of senior nursing-management positions. Many took early retirement.

As an educator, I was asked to accompany four of the orthopedic surgeons to another hospital to help develop staff skills to deliver health care focusing on this group of clients. The move went smoothly, and would you believe that within one year, that hospital was merging with two others.

I assisted with the transformation and then applied for a job opportunity to teach in a long-term care home. I had the choice and the courage to move into another area of nursing.

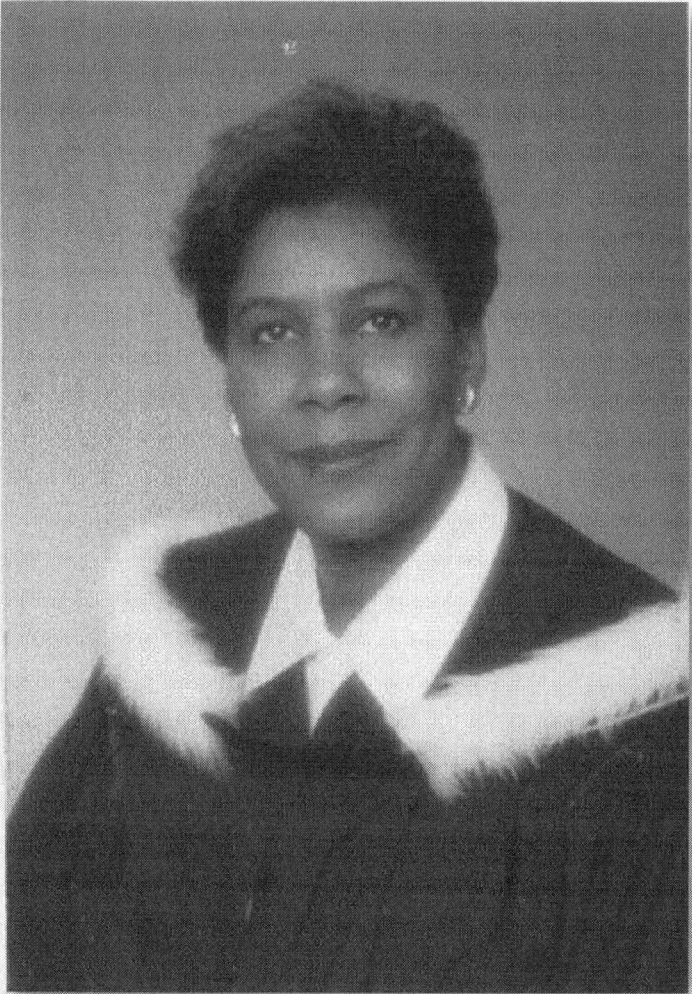

BA Graduate, University of Toronto

# CHAPTER 4

# Leadership Role in Long-Term Care: Supervisor Education

~c~

*My greatest memory of you in nursing is when you*
*were working at Kipling Long-Term Care Home as*
*our staff educator. You were one great teacher who*
*saw the best in everyone and would take time out*
*make each person feel valued. The impact you left*
*on me was seeing my capabilities, and enrolled me to*
*get additional training to provide more effective and*
*loving healthcare for our seniors. Wow! I so enjoyed*
*learning new skills, such as understanding how to*
*deliver care including families that were so worried*
*and needed guidance on better care approaches*
*for the residents who had dementia. Thanks.*

—*RPN,* Long-Term Care Home

JUST WHEN I THOUGHT I would continue my nursing career working in an acute-care hospital, an opportunity was presented to me to teach in a different setting. I had increased my nursing expertise to the point where I felt I could work in any health-care environment. It was an easy decision to make as hospital mergers were in full force, and educators were sent wherever the conglomerates decided.

I also wanted to obtain a master's degree in adult education, and moving into this new role provided me with research opportunities and a bit more downtime to complete my thesis. I was so blessed; I had not failed any job interview I had undertaken. This interview was special, being the first where seniors who resided in a long-term care home participated.

I was floored by two questions the seniors asked, and I took my time to think very carefully about my responses.

"Miss Nicholson, some of the nurses get upset when I ask if I can learn how to use the computer. They respond that there is no computer for the residents, so the training cannot happen. As our new educator, how would you help us to learn to use the computer?" asked an elderly resident.

"I love the idea that you want to learn about computers. Give me some time to find out what we need to do together to make this happen," I responded. A broad smile spread across his face, and he thanked me.

"The nurses do a good job, the best they can. What difference would an educator make?" asked the second resident.

I got brave and asked a question instead of answering. *"Tell me one thing that would make life more fun to live in your home."*

"Having more music in my life," he said. I encouraged him to meet with me once the interview was completed, and we would talk about specific ways to make this happen.

I was so excited to be engaged in an interview where seniors' participation was valued. Right away, I felt at home in this new role, knowing I would be sharing my expertise with staff and all the residents.

Orientation to my role as an educator in this setting was quite different from any I had participated in before. There were ten long-term care homes that belonged to the city; all new employees received orientation at one of the homes where there was classroom space. As a new educator, I was asked to facilitate discussions on managing a library system and enhancing the care for residents who have Alzheimer's disease.

What more could an educator ask for? I was the president of the Alzheimer Society of our region, and I also managed the community library where staff and family of that organization accessed the resources. I participated in aspects of orientation with frontline staff. We discussed fire safety, working with all levels of staff, residents, volunteers, families, and the other health-care sectors such as hospitals and other long-term care homes.

I gave the administrator of the home a list of other orientation activities in which I would participate, including those I would access on my own. I planned meetings with each manager to hear firsthand their education needs and that of their staff. I attended staff and residents' meetings to hear directly from them in order to develop education plans. The city also has legislations on annual education where staff must be recertified or retrained. I quickly reviewed the poli-cy and procedure manuals to aid my planning. I traveled to the other nine homes and met with my colleagues, who were full-time and part-time educators. We bonded as we shared unique ways of helping all stakeholders be successful.

A memorable aspect of orientation I planned to ac-cess myself was learning about the daily care the residents required and what methods were used. I requested permis-sion from the unit managers to work alongside the personal-support workers so that I could get to know them and also observe some of their educational requirements. These are the groups of health-care workers in the homes who do most of the hands-on care and work the hardest.

Managers granted permission and assisted in commu-nicating this request to the staff at their monthly meetings. This was not an approach previously seen by any of the staff, and they verbalized fear I would be interacting with them only to incorrectly criticize what they were doing. However, I made my schedule to align with theirs for four weeks and was on duty in my scrubs daily at either 0700 hours or 1500 hours when there was a change of tours. I explained to the personal-support workers that I need them to educate me about their jobs, so I gain a better understanding of their challenges and was then able to help them gain enhanced skills.

I worked alongside each personal-support worker; met the residents; and assisted with all aspects of care such as hy-giene, bathing, bed making, and feeding those who were un-able to do so. I became an intricate part of the team while at the same time encouraging them to try other ways of getting their work done. I reminded them daily of how valuable they were to the residents, their families, and their workplace. I purposefully did not mention any negatives except where there were urgent safety issues. Instead of saying a task was done wrong, I offered to help make their work safer and provided an even safer environment for the residents.

The good news spread among the four hundred staff in the long-term care home.

"Norma, I am sorry for what I told others you would probably do. I thought you were coming to pick on what we're doing and tell our managers we were not doing a good job; instead, you helped us to learn better ways of working safer. We are so thankful to you and hope you stay to help us more," said one personal-support worker.

Seeing the good outcomes for one level of their staff, managers started making appointments to have discussions with me about managing their staff. Some staff were seen as lazy, others as slow and functioning below expectations. The workload for all staff who worked in a long-term care home was heavy, and I sensed the managers were tired and did not have much success in motivating their staff to do more.

What an opportunity to support these folks, and also to carry out my master's degree thesis about leadership! I also spent every waking hour planning to help the managers.

A manager, when asked if she wished to say something about my interaction with her while I worked in the facility as an educator, said, "Something that impacted my life is your calm manner in which you handled any and every situation, and always saw the positive in any given situation. There was a time when I was experiencing a very challenging time with a certain staff and you helped me to see it was not about me. That staff was going through a difficult time at home, was not coping, and brought that baggage to the workplace. You suggested you would sit in with me if the staff allowed this and would be present only to listen, take notes, and assist with follow-up.

"When we met with the nurse, she unloaded all her frustrations and 'not knowing how to get help.' You sat in that meeting, smiled, nodded, and said nothing! I was so encouraged, and the nurse welcomed the discussion. You even sat with the nurse after, made her a cup of tea, and offered to meet with her to set up counseling sessions for her. I was a happier manager, and my staff was much happier and a joy to have in the workplace."

I organized my workday to ensure my interactions and education outreach to all levels of staff was what they had requested to grow. Would you believe that housekeeping and dietary staff came to seek my help around continuing education? After one year as the educator in the home, four former housekeeping staff returned to school part-time and graduated from the personal-support worker program.

On my to-do list were the following items for follow up, planning, and execution in my first year:

* Requests from the residents who participated in my interview.

- Developing a leadership program in collaboration with the senior team, managers, and the educators in the other homes.
- Assist staff in identifying their educational needs, which should align with working more effectively and carrying out self-care.
- Collaborate with all stakeholders to assist with decreasing sick and absent days, ensuring increased productivity.

Permission was obtained from the senior team to facilitate and educate high school co-ops, personal-support workers, and nursing students. With the help of other educators in the long-term care homes, relationships were developed with the various educational institutions regarding student placements and the processes for them to be effective.

There was always a bit of resistance from frontline staff when so many students would be invading their workspace. With the help of senior registered nurses and teachers from the education facilities, we developed the processes ensuring a great learning environment and ways to motivate and reward the staff for their engagement. There was transparency and effective communication with all the staff to ensure understanding of the role of each category of students. To ensure effective flow of these new arrangements, each category of students was approved in three-month intervals. There were a few times when there was overlap of co-op students with nursing students, but both groups quickly learned the roles of each other.

I ensured that the physicians, interdisciplinary team, residents, and families were informed about student activities and provided opportunities to respond to concerns from all of these groups. The nurses were so happy to include students in daily activities; after a while, they began to say, "This is my student." Positive changes occurred quickly in the home, and staff met often to discuss and resolve issues. One could see the change in the environment, and staff actually wanted to be at work. There was no urgency to act on a plan for increasing attendance. We had several graduations for the different groups of students. Many personal-support worker students returned to work full or part time after their graduation.

The many ways in which students enhanced the lives of residents:

- Enhanced socialization by reading, walking, playing board games, or just sitting with a resident to watch TV, ensuring the resident did not become lonely.
- Taught residents basic computer programs, such as e-mails and writing simple documents. (Who says folks who are experiencing dementia cannot learn new ideas? A majority of these residents proved this to be a myth.)
- Assisted with many aspects of adding joy to enjoying meal times. Students were taught safe feeding and assisting residents in safe ways.
- Accompanied the residents to the gift shop, library, and social gatherings in the home.

♦ Participated in recreation programs facilitated by the staff of that service.

♦ Residents, who were unable to get out of bed, verbalized their appreciation of having the students assist them in similar ways.

I was granted the go-ahead to carry out my research and titled my thesis, "Evaluating the Outcomes of a Nursing Leadership Training in a Long-Term Care Facility."

The purpose of the study was to determine whether the training of registered nursing staff in skills to lead their team enabled them to become effective leaders in the workplace. The study was carried out over three months post training to give time for the implementation of new guided practices in the workplace. It involved two groups of nurses: those who participated in an eighteen-hour six-module leadership training and those who were nonparticipants. It was mandatory that all managers participate in the training and the follow-up requirements. They were responsible for facilitating short meetings each week with their team to identify what was going well and where they needed the educator's assistance to manage issues.

The purpose of the study was fourfold:

1. Has the training assisted them to lead their team more effectively?
2. Are there gaps in the sustainability of the acquired skills?

3. What leadership skills do nonparticipants practice?
4. What are the ongoing learning needs of nursing leaders?

A survey was used to obtain their responses regarding the outcome of the training and impact on their team. The nonparticipants also completed a questionnaire where they were asked about the differences seen in colleagues who had attended the training. Their observations were similar to those who participated in the training: those who participated had developed added abilities to problem-solve and work collaboratively with their team. The managers verbalized that they felt they were now employed in an active learning environment and felt more capable to lead.

Outcomes from all participants:

- Effective leaders must be lifelong learners.
- The leader must have quick thinking and fast action.
- Leaders must have the ability to think critically, solve problems, respect people, communicate skillfully, and set specific goals to develop themselves and others.
- Learning does not always take place in a classroom setting.

Based on the outcome of this leadership training, recommendations were made to ensure annual need assessments that would aid in future education, with processes in place to sustain the new skills and the integration of the training into the leaders' performance appraisals.

Our personal development was often steered by our careers, our workplaces, and our jobs. It could sometimes feel as if our work was pulling us along, forcing us to learn things and develop skills in areas that do not fit into our deepest interests. These employees wanted to learn and kept their minds open to possibilities. Their learning and engagement were designed around what they wanted to learn, and being able to use the information benefited many stakeholders.

We worked hard to implement and sustain the training. There were monthly evaluations to assess if the new skills acquired during the training were being utilized, in order to identify any gaps for enhanced training. The registered nurses who participated in the training were supported in mentoring other nurses, and together we developed small focus groups of the leaders to discuss any problems or challenges that came about during implementation. Participants verbalized that doing the training was fun, but some parts were difficult to implement since not all the staff were of the same category, and each delivered different levels of care.

Many other opportunities for interaction and education came my way in this long-term-care home. I delivered education to the residents, volunteers, and families who were able to participate.

I organized workshops for frontline staff and partnered with their managers to assign specific time off for them to attend. I researched community-education opportunities for all levels of staff, ensuring senior management and frontline staff attended a minimum of one workshop or conference annually.

I loved to bake. I had a small education budget, and I was therefore able to purchase ingredients to bake so that the staff who attended weekly thirty-minute education sessions always had snacks while they were learning.

I provided coverage for educators in the other city homes when they were on vacation or on lengthy sick leave. I did this by facilitating orientation of new staff, and I visited the homes to assess and support staff education.

My work life changed when there were no longer any maintenance employees on the weekend working in this home. I routinely worked one weekend day each month, Saturday or Sunday. With budgetary cutbacks, I did not have the opportunity to carry out only teaching on the weekend for the part-time staff who did not work in the week. I became the manager on the weekend, and I was responsible for all aspects of care and safety in the home.

When an elevator stopped working, and there was no maintenance staff on site, I would try to get it started up again or close it until Monday morning. When the large dishwasher broke and the dishes from breakfast were not washed for dinner, I was responsible for organizing paper ware and some items that were tools to aid safe eating for residents. I had to go to the kitchen and wash these special eating aids for the residents.

The staff, residents, families, and visitors would be disgruntled and insisted I make the necessary changes, such as getting someone in to fix the elevator. There were three elevators; the service one was used for transportation of items such as linen and wheelchairs, and two were used for residents, staff, and visitors. If the service elevator was broken, then there would be only one in use for others, which caused backups and slow movement.

I requested changes to these processes and received the same responses: "We no longer have a budget to have people here doing nothing on the weekend or to be called in at overtime pay."

After three years, I gave my notice to leave this wonderful work environment, where I had fallen in love with so many residents and staff.

At my good-bye reception, a manager said, "Norma, people will forget what you said, they will forget what you did, but they will never forget how you made them feel."

I gained so much education and built many levels of relationships that continue to impact the way I interact with seniors and their families today. I am reminded that someone who has Alzheimer's disease has a beautiful heart; the disease is what has changed who that person was.

I continue to use community opportunities to teach and support those who are struggling with this disease.

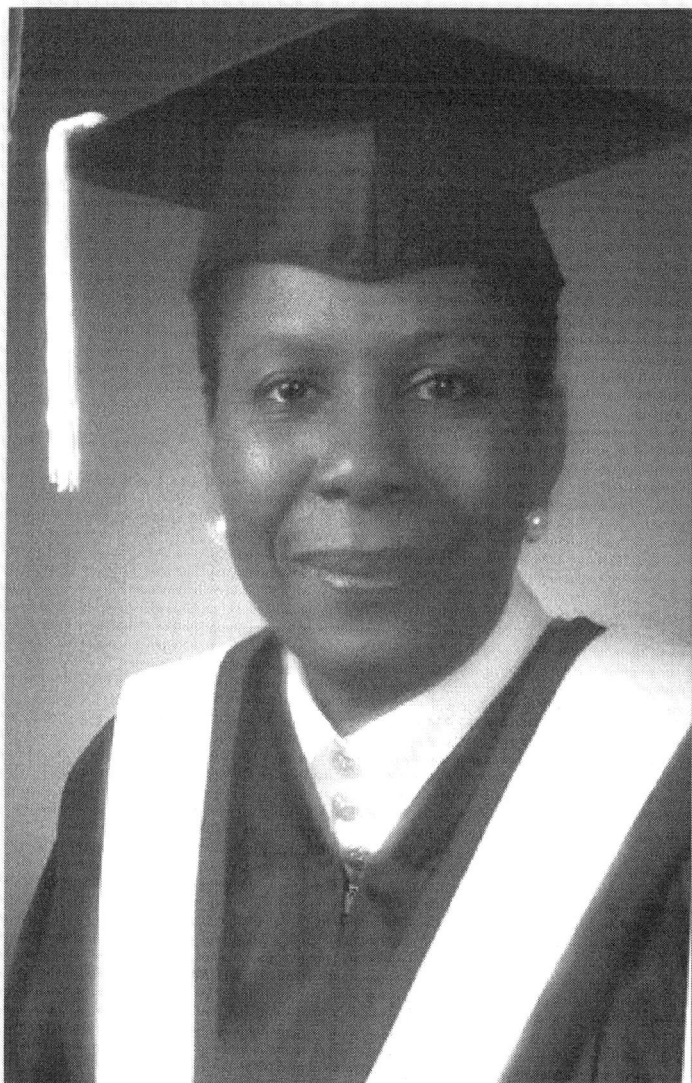

MA Graduate, Central Michigan

# CHAPTER 5

# Leadership in Ambulatory Rehabilitation: Manager

Whenever I find myself doubting how far I can go, I try to remember how far I have come. I recall the many challenges I have faced, all the battles I have won, and all the fears I have overcome.

I take 100 percent responsibility for what happens to my nursing career, being fully aware that some failures come from taking risks. I know success happens when preparation meets opportunities.

I worked in a variety of health-care sectors as manager and educator, and continuously increased my education. With these combined skills, I have this unique opportunity to reflect on past work environments where I had the choice of staying or moving to another.

I decided to move to a work environment in which I had not previously worked, not only for the skills I would gain but for the opportunity to enhance my knowledge and interact with patients who were mainly seeking rehabilitation while living in their communities.

With my team of interdisciplinary staff, I managed thirteen patient-centered care areas under this portfolio. We engaged in many innovative, evidenced-based methods to enhance and advance quality of care for our outpatients.

I think that this rehab facility was the first to carry out research and application of the drug, Botox, to enhance the lives of poststroke patients. In this setting, there was also a focus on using innovative care approaches to help those who had postpolio syndrome; by using hydrotherapy, they were now able to live happier lives.

Many dynamic changes were occurring in this work environment, most of which I supported, especially the increased access to computers to support scheduling of patients and to complete documentation in a timely manner. However, I was not supportive of the changes to programs that would negatively impact the lives of elderly patients receiving rehabilitation for chronic conditions, such as strokes, postpolio, and major motor-vehicle accidents.

Nurses can be public activists and advocates; it is assumed we are free to bring up questions about the quality of care the public should expect from their health-care system and providers. In some settings, when in the role of a manager, you do as you are told by the administration.

I walked through the ambulatory clinic one morning and observed an elderly gentleman sitting in a wheelchair looking quite sad. Looking at the time, I realized that it was 8:30 a.m. and only the clerk was in the department. The multidisciplinary team worked flexible tours of duty to meet the needs of patients, and I knew none would be in the department until 9:00 a.m.

I walked toward the patient, asked if I could sit on the chair next to him, and introduced myself as the manager for the department. I apologized that he had arrived so early when there was no staff to assist him. Mr. B informed me that Wheel-Trans brought him, and he had no choice but to arrive at that time, though his appointment was not until 9:00 a.m. I offered to purchase a cup of coffee for him and went to the cafeteria to do so. I returned with a coffee for him and one for myself. We talked for a while longer, and during the conversation, I asked if we could have someone in the department earlier to facilitate his therapy on his arrival. Would he be able to arrange a return by Wheel-Trans right after?

In my nursing career, this is the second time I had seen someone's smile spread fully across his face. The first time I saw this reaction was as a volunteer; I sat with a patient and read many areas of the sports section of the paper. He had been in the hospital for several months, without a TV and without his glasses, which were left at his home. He was unable to obtain any updates on his favorite sports. His happiness shone through.

Mr. B said that sometimes, when Wheel-Trans returned for him, he had to leave before his hydrotherapy was completed, and it would be good if I could make this change. I knew one of my physiotherapy staff would love to start working at 8:00 a.m. due to childcare responsibilities. I promised to phone the patient with the follow-up after having a discussion with the team in the department. They supported their colleagues, and also thought of one other patient who would like to come earlier for hydrotherapy. This was a win-win for the staff and the patients.

I engaged the staff and the clerk to inform the patients and make the changes to their ambulatory schedules. The following week, while working in the office, my staff physiotherapist came and knocked on the door. She asked if I could take a few minutes to come to the department to speak with Mr. B. I sensed there was something exciting to be seen.

"Norma, you're going to be surprised!"

On entering the department, I noticed Mr. B seated in his wheelchair; he was waving his arm to direct me to the pool area. He had asked his physiotherapist to gather all staff to come to that area. After I said good morning to everyone, Mr. B asked if he could donate $25,000 to renovate our pool.

"What did you say? You're giving us that much money?" I asked. Before saying thanks, I asked the clerk to page a member from our senior management team and our foundation to come to the department.

Mr. B shared with us that he owned a large commercial outlet from which we purchased all our office supplies, and he could also ensure that we receive a year's donation of these supplies.

Even today, when I think of what positive changes can occur if we only validate and respect each other, I constantly give, expecting nothing in return. Had I walked by this patient and only said hello, I do not think this magic would have happened.

On the arrival of a senior manager and the CEO of the hospital foundation, Mr. B repeated his offer.

When asked why, he said, "The manager and staff of this department have valued me, they really care, and now I must give back."

I openly shed tears, and I noticed many of my staff were also crying. What an impact we had made on this person's life, without even knowing the potential returns.

The hospital foundation took care of obtaining the dollars, and followed up with engaging the patient and staff regarding the changes to the pool area. Within one year of receiving the donation, contractors had completed the renovation to the hydrotherapy pool and change rooms. In the *Mississauga News*, one of the weekend headlines read, "Norma Nicholson Poses by the Facility Rehabilitation Pool, Which Is Her Pride and Joy."

Many pictures were taken at the formal reopening of this beautiful area, and this change positively impacted all staff, visitors, volunteers, and patients.

You have followed me through my career thus far and know that ongoing learning is one of my values. I strived to instill the same in all my staff and, where possible, encourage them by paying for courses or workshops, giving a paid day to attend, or even encouraging them to use a vacation day when the cost of the workshop was expensive and I was paying. For those who did not get to attend, I encouraged those who attended to return and share their knowledge with colleagues.

The director of education approved a two-day workshop for me. I wanted to learn more about the new computers being installed and to teach and support the staff with these changes. I was happy to obtain approval, and I attended the education session in another facility on a Monday and Tuesday.

I returned to work at 8:00 a.m. on Wednesday morning, excited to share what I had learned with my director and my staff. I planned to go around my departments to visit staff, but on my way to the first department, I received a page to come to the human-resources department.

I went to the fifth floor in the other building and walked into the office of the director of human resources. Something felt unusual.

She came forward and said, "Do come in and have a seat. We've been paging you since 8:00 a.m."

I did not respond as I found this encounter unusual. I was invited further into her office, where I found my director standing by the window. I thought something terrible had occurred to a patient or one of my staff during my absence.

I was informed my services would be terminated without cause. It did not matter that my performance review two months earlier demonstrated I was "a very effective nursing leader" and "patient-satisfaction surveys were at their high-est"; the decision was made to terminate and not provide me with a reason why my employment was no longer required.

Stunned and dismayed, I did not ask why. I asked if I could make a phone call, and I called my husband to come and take me home.

"Are you ill?" was his first question. "You drove to work a short while ago."

I informed him that a half hour ago, I had a job, and now I did not; therefore, I was dazed and unable to drive home.

Neither the human-resources director nor my nursing director sat at the table with me. The human-resources director stretched her hands toward me and handed me a brown envelope.

"Read and sign these documents when you're home, and call us if you have any questions," she said. She requested the return of my keys and pager. This meant I would not be able to return to my office to get my purse or any of my belongings.

It was a cool September morning. The leaves were beginning to lose their chlorophyll and, looking out the window from the fifth floor where this department was located, I could also see the beam of the sun over the horizon. This was my reality; I had just been terminated from my job.

In a daze, I walked toward the stairs on the fifth floor. I was afraid if I took the elevator, I would meet someone who might ask why I was crying. My eyes flooded with burning tears at the thought of being unemployed, of leaving what I loved to do. I ran down the stairs to meet my husband outside the building.

Reaching the last step of the winding stairway, I pushed the door to open it, only to find—due to security measures—it was locked, and I had no keys. I sat on the step for a while until I heard footsteps behind me; looking up, I saw the manager of another department, who stated he was asked to find me as my spouse had arrived. He had also brought my purse, but none of my other belongings.

I shivered as I exited the door; the coat I had worn that morning had not been retrieved from my office. Losing my job in this manner was painful, but the stress that grew out of this dismissal was that there was no opportunity to say goodbye to my staff. My husband drove me home. I was so happy he was able to do this as the tears continued to flow; I would not have been able to see my way.

About one mile from home, a police officer pulled us over and explained we were driving over the speed limit. I informed the officer I was a nurse and had just been fired from my job, and I was so sorry we were not obeying the law. I explained my husband was also upset, and he may not have been paying close attention to the speed at which we were traveling. I promised we would abide by the law as we continued to drive.

The officer told me he was the father of a premature infant who had lived at the children's hospital since birth. Every day, he overheard the nurses say they did not have an adequate number of nurses to provide care to these infants.

He further elaborated that, being a nurse, I had many opportunities open for me, but I could eliminate them if I caused an accident while driving. I thanked him for his kindness and waved good-bye, quite relieved we were not issued a ticket.

He directed us to wait until he was able to get us back on the street safely, as we needed to reverse the vehicle first. I looked toward the back of the vehicle as my husband reversed.

"Where's the police officer?" I asked. We were both surprised there was no officer directing us on the roadway, because he had disappeared.

This event remains vivid in my mind to this day. I do believe in angels, and I know an angel saved us from a terrible accident. My tears went away; I felt sad, but a very warm feeling came over my whole being, and I felt I would find another job.

I contacted the human-resources department and requested a date and time to retrieve my personal belongings. In the company of my husband, the human-resources director, and a security guard, I took all my belongings and did not turn back.

Many of my staff could not work the day of my termination. They told me it was like a dream where they wanted to wake up from a nightmare. I received phone calls from them every day, even on the weekends on their days off. Many gathered at my home and brought me good-bye gifts. I felt at peace, because I had overcome many challenges before. One of the clerks from my departments brought me a note that read:

You have inspired people to do their best by building a life of trust by your day-to-day interactions;
keep loving your life of ministering to others.

With the help of friends, family, and my church, I decided
to rest for three months before starting a job search. I tried
to think positive, but in my mind, I created an inner critic
of being a failure and became ashamed of losing my job. I
was mentored and coached into turning my inner critic into
an inner coach. I was able to stop feeling like a failure, and I
started engaging in activities to lift me up.

Mentors do not like to have their time wasted. I had a
close relationship with my mentor; I was comfortable asking
questions, and I acted with positive energy.

"If God shuts a door, stop banging on it. Trust that whatever is behind it is not meant for you. Every time you think
you are being rejected from something good, you are being
redirected to something better." I repeated this several times
to myself, which made me stronger.

# CHAPTER 6

# Helping Troubled Youth Turn Their Lives Around

ی

*What we do not see, what most of us never*
*suspect of existing, is the silent but irresistible*
*power which comes to the rescue of those who*
*fight on in the face of discouragement.*

—*Napoleon Hill*

Chances are that many managers in organizations will face termination without cause. As mergers, downsizing, and increased technology lead to a decreased number of employees, some are turfed out of their work environment. How you accept these sudden notices without discouragement is most important to your mental health.

Negative thoughts can come at you with such speed; you can become overwhelmed with managing the outcomes. Did you know each of us, as adults, have sixty thousand thoughts per day? Most of these thoughts are negative. I learned how to talk to myself as a winner. Today, I am where my positive thoughts have brought me, and I know there are unlimited possibilities when one remains positive. I am not saying I have not experienced times when I felt discouraged; however, these thoughts are inconveniences, not insurmountable barriers.

After a short period of hibernation, goal planning, and attending a few conferences, it was time to seek new employment. My mentors had encouraged and helped enhance my confidence to face new situations.

In my online job search, I came across the Charity Village, where I found a job opportunity for a nurse to develop, design, and manage health care in a large, secure youth-custody setting. I had not worked in the criminal-youth justice system, but thinking of possibilities, I felt I could do this job well.

Henry Ford said, "Whether you think you can or think you can't—you're right."

The application and interview processes were superb. At the end of the interview, I thanked the panel and gave my list of references to the human-resources personnel. In my heart and mind, I knew this job belonged to me. I would have been left with doubts if my references were not readily accepted. I headed home, having been told I would be informed about the decision in a few days.

Within four hours of participating in the interview, the phone rang. My heart skipped a beat; I hesitated to pick up the receiver, but noticed the number displayed was connected to the human-resources department. I was offered the job of health-care manager in a large 192-bed youth-custody facility. I celebrated with some of my former staff and with family and friends. What a joy to turn over a new leaf.

There was a brand-new work setting—the grounds for the buildings were just being prepared. A small number of us were employed to develop, design, and implement specific services for incarcerated youth. I had great opportunities to collaborate with stakeholders, such as families, volunteers, physicians, nurses, and community-support teams.

An experienced registered nurse was assigned to work with me to develop policies and procedures and to design a youth-focused health-care system. I knew from news media and my volunteer work in the community that many of the youth incarcerated in Ontario—and other areas in the world, too—are black males.

I had great compassion and empathy for marginalized and underserved youth and their families. The circumstances surrounding my childhood and youth could have projected me into areas of crime—born into abject poverty, suffering unspeakable and horrific abuses, plus abandonment, could have formed that basis. Due to my grandmother's love and gaining higher education and guidance from mentors and coaches, I had skills and life experiences to engage stakeholders in managing the health of those youth.

I became highly engaged in community planning to ensure a variety of health-care personnel to deliver youth-focused care in a custody facility. Job postings went out, guided by human resources; many interviews occurred, and the right individuals were selected for different areas of care. The team consisted of registered nurses, psychiatrists, medical doctors, a dentist, optometrist, and physiotherapist.

Partnerships were built with community agencies, such as physiotherapists, pharmacists, and occupational therapists. Internal partnerships were formed with social workers and psychologists to ensure holistic health care was delivered.

In building a new team and learning the roles in a secure-custody facility, I encouraged all employees to take responsibility for their performance through open communication and realistic goal setting.

I ensured our team had resources and opportunities for learning, and I involved them in problem-solving and decision-making.

I communicated what we needed to have in place before opening day; I explained the benefits of taking responsibilities for the youth's input in an environment where previous skills were highly valued. We were afforded several months to prepare before the youth were transferred to the facility.

Our health-care department replicated many family-health-care clinics in the community, and the youth had daily access to care. We designed wonderful youth-focused health-care rooms with modern equipment; we developed schedules for the staff and the youth, along with policies and procedures around processes. Emergency-only care was provided for the staff.

A youth who experienced emergency-health-care needs in the absence of a nurse would be securely transferred to hospital in the community. Should surgery or a period of admission be required, the youth would be admitted with a staff member to ensure a safe and secure environment.

Some of my nursing colleagues asked me about the role of a registered nurse in "jail." This was a great opportunity to educate them about youth caught up in the justice system and what nurses and other multidisciplinary team members could do to help them stay healthy, return to optimal health, and learn about health maintenance.

Incarcerated youth experience similar health-care needs as all of us in our communities. They could present with mental-health challenges, uncontrolled diabetes, chronic pain, or respiratory and infectious diseases. Nurses had to have the skills, compassion, and caring approach used in all health-care practices. In fact, as the manager who visited the youth daily in their cottages or saw them in the health-care department, it was not important to me what charges brought them to this setting. I was more concerned about their health and the way we delivered care in a respectful, sensitive, and caring manner.

When I assisted the nurses in carrying out admission of a new youth, I learned so much during those private and confidential conversations. I truly feel in my heart that if our society would come alongside youth and families struggling with aspects of their lives, we would not need jails for our youth.

## Two Examples Readily Come to Mind

John, a youth, presented with frequent need to manage his anger, sometimes engaged in fights with others and was brought over to the segregation room. John had spent the night in this area of the facility and remained quite angry the following morning. His name was placed on the schedule to see the medical doctor, but he refused to leave the room. One of the nursing staff asked for my assistance, as it was very important that John not miss his appointment to hear the results of an X-ray.

I went to the area, and I respectfully requested the youth-service officers allow me to speak with John. They responded that he was very angry and would not want to talk with me. However, at my insistence, they opened the door. The youth was lying in bed. I called him by his name and asked if I could enter the room.

"What for?" he said.

I informed him the doctor was in the health-care department and wanted to see him.

"What for?" he asked again. I asked his permission to come closer to his bed, and he said, "Yes, ma'am."

As I got closer to his bed, he sat up facing me, and I smiled. I told him my name, my role, and that I would really like him to see the doctor. I asked if he recalled the X-ray they had taken two days prior; he said yes. I told him the result was abnormal, and we needed to privately discuss his options for treatment.

*"I'll come now,"* he responded. I was so proud of him. I thanked John for agreeing to see the doctor and told him the youth-services officers would take him to the department.

When he arrived to see the doctor and the nurse, I again asked permission to be in the treatment room where he was being seen. He had a chronic respiratory disease and required medication to remain healthy. This was explained, along with the side effects, and he was told the nurse would ensure the medication was given to him each day. All his anger dissipated—someone cared about him and his health. He had lived in his community, and he was not diagnosed until he was incarcerated. I found this so sad.

Justin, another male youth in the facility, had refused to attend school. He was not attending school prior to being incarcerated. He told everyone he did not do well in school and he was afraid to go, and therefore it was a waste of time for him. Justin was given an opportunity to start school in his room, where a teacher would visit to assist him. He did not complete his assignments, and his behavior declined as he was forced to attend school. It was mandatory for all incarcerated youth to attend school, unless they had a medical reason for temporary absences.

Justin was scheduled to visit the health-care department to have an assessment by the optometrist. His vision was greatly decreased, and he had not told anyone he was having a problem seeing. Perhaps he had gotten used to a darkened world. The nurses ordered eyeglasses for him, and when they were available, he was accompanied to the health-care department to meet with the optometrist.

Justin took his glasses from the optometrist, placed them on his face, walked around in the room, and said, "Oh shit—my God—the wall is white, and the floor is level."

"What are you talking about?" the optometrist asked.

"This was the same room, man. I came in to get my blood work, and the walls and floor were different colors," he responded. He now realized how much of his sight he had lost.

A small miracle happened: Justin started to attend school five days per week, did all his assignments, and was so motivated by his progress that he wrote a letter to the health-care team thanking them for their support. When youth or families were experiencing poverty, the health-care department undertook the purchase of glasses for them. We were honored to help with the purchase of eyeglasses for this youth to assist him in moving forward in life.

There were a few situations over which we had no control, but they had a negative reflection on our health-care team. It took patience and open and transparent communication to guide effective follow-up.

An Example

A youth diagnosed with a mental illness was admitted to custody at midnight and had an early appointment to go to court the following morning. He received breakfast before leaving and was escorted to a court located some distance from the facility. A nurse did not see him, as no nurses were on site between midnight and 6:00 a.m. Youth in the facility would be escorted to community health care if an overnight emergency occurred.

On the nurses' arrival to the department each day, they planned to complete health-care admissions for youth who were not seen on their last tour of duty. This youth's name was on the list to be admitted, but he had left early for court. The department's main phone rang at 9:30 a.m., and a nurse transferred the call to my office, requesting I facilitate a discussion with a parent who had asked to speak with the manager for the department. It was the mother of the youth who had left for court. She informed me she was at the court, and her son told her he had not received his morning medications.

I began to apologize for this and to provide an explanation, but the mother began shouting in explicit and disrespectful language over the phone. I thought I knew a bit of street language, but I had not heard some of these before. When she stopped to take a breath, I informed her that should her son return after his court appointment, we would ensure he received his medication.

I can still feel a tremor running throughout my body when I reflect on the tone and language used by this mother. This interaction led me to wonder what kind of home environment the youth came from. He received bail at the court and did not return to custody, and I had no opportunity to meet the youth or his parent.

"Helping Troubled Youth Turn Their Lives Around" was the headline in the *Toronto Star* in April 2010, two years after I began working as the manager. In response to the call for

Nightingale Nurses nominations, a third-year nursing student nominated me as a great nursing leader for this recognition.

"Very few nursing leaders would set out to provide health care for youth who have been at risk, have actually committed crimes, and are housed in secure custody. These youth are not seen as having made a mistake, but are viewed very negatively by our society," she stated when she spoke with the reporter.

I had been recognized with four previous annual Nightingale Certificates, but this, the fifth, was an honorable mention in the Toronto Star Nightingale Awards of 2010. Excited yet humble, I reflected on how I was moved to apply for a health-care manager's role in the largest youth secure-custody facility in the province.

A quote from Louise Hays came to mind, because of the way my previous employment ended:

It is relatively easy to feel grateful when good things are happening and life is going the way we want it to. Even then, we often take things for granted. It is interesting, though, that after going through difficult times, in retrospect we can often see that there was something important and necessary about that experience.

During the same time, another headline blazed from the event program for the Eighteenth Annual Scholarship Awards

Ball of Black Law Enforcers (ABLE): "From the Corridors of Hospitals: Building Healthcare for Youth in a Security-Custody Environment."

The article provided readers with an overview of how I had impacted major changes in our society through being a registered nurse. It further stated I was a compassionate, caring mentor grounded in my professional values, and a great nursing leader who was being recognized for my work with students and new immigrants.

I was very grateful for this organization and its members.

I am a nursing alumnus of a wonderful college, George Brown College, and was recognized in their community news for my work within a secure youth-custody facility. In 2009, in their Community Online News Section, the college wrote the headline "Nurse rises to the final challenge of a 30-year career as an outstanding professional": "She has undertaken probably one of the most challenging posts to date…that of designing and developing health-care services for 192 youth in one of the largest secure youth-custody facilities dedicated to service young people who are in conflict with the law." With mixed emotions, I retired from my employment in the youth criminal-justice system in 2012. I promised myself that I would continue to advocate for marginalized and under-served youth in my community. I was now able to connect with some of the community groups that deliver support to youth post incarceration. Remember that mother who spoke so harshly on the phone in a conversation about her son who was incarcerated; I plan to go into communities and seek safe spaces to educate parents about managing challenging behavior of their teenagers before they become involved with the criminal-justice system. What a joy and a profound experience it was to be highly engaged in the health care of incarcerated youth, ages twelve to seventeen years! This is the job where I learned the most and underwent the most challenges in my nursing career. I would not have changed anything.

All is well with me, and God hears my words and makes them come true. One day, none of our children and youth will be incarcerated, as we will build a world to help them reach their potential.

Please show your children love; value them each day of their lives.

CHAPTER 7

# Enjoying Community Volunteer Work In My Retirement

———⟋⟍———

MOHAMMED ALI SAID, SERVICE TO others is the rent you pay for your room here on earth. I have a passion for serving others and as I grew older and transitioned into retirement, I became more aware that the two hands I have, one is for helping others and the other for helping myself.

I cannot envision staying at home every day after going to work five days weekly for over forty years. How boring that would be!

Forty years ago, I began enquiry into a nursing profession after I became a volunteer in an adult hospital setting. That opportunity allowed me to gain access to my dream career serving others and growing in leaps and bounds. It is a 360- degree turn to now see myself as a retiree and enjoying and participating in several different volunteer roles. I remain highly motivated to help others but this time there is the added bonus of what I gain such as getting out of the house, meeting new folks, learning about different cultural needs, developing new friends, gaining new knowledge and sharing my skills.

I have the ability to work willingly with others for the betterment of my community. Donating my time and energy is a very meaningful experience for me as well as the organizations in which I am involved.

I sometimes hear folks say that volunteering is just doing something nice, however I know from personal experiences that the volunteer work that I do have great impact on my community.

I have a passion for seeing the good in everyone no matter what their lived experiences have been and I convey caring through my words and actions. I remain very humble throughout my life and do understand that I cannot live the experiences of another person but I can get alongside them and help to lift them up out certain situations using the skills and knowledge that I have gained.

Volunteering in a Variety of Organizations
Youth Shelter:

What are some factors that lead to homelessness for young persons? You are 16 years old and sleeping on a parked bench when a police officer drives by and see you sleeping outside. You will be asked where are your parents and your home, and on responding that you are homeless, most often you will be directed to a youth shelter and you are documented as being homeless.  There are many reasons why young people become homeless. There are wonderful family units and there are many dysfunctional ones who do not support their adolescents to pursue meaningful goals to reach the potential they are capable of.

A young person can run away from home due to the dysfunction he or she has been experiencing. There may be domestic violence, parents who have addictions to drugs and alcohol, experiencing mental health issues themselves and living in abject poverty where the young person is not provided with the necessities of life. Research has shown that most youth run away from home due to neglect and abuse. This abuse can be physical, sexual or emotional or a combination of all three forms.

Covenant House, a youth shelter reports that about 40% of the youth seen by their service providers identify as lesbians, gay, bisexual or transgender. They are literally kicked out of their homes as some parents say this is a chosen lifestyle. They do not take the time to listen and help the young person. There are those who become homeless when they exit the child welfare and the criminal youth justice systems and have no consistent support or are unaware of ways to seek help. Others face mental illness and the behaviour they demonstrate cannot be dealt with at home so they choose to live on the street. A few families may reach out to help but for the vast majority of youth going home is not an option. Most need help from community agencies and service providers to find permanents homes and meaningful lives.

I use my human resources skills and knowledge to assist homeless youth rise above unemployment. I had been driving by this beautiful home in my neighbourhood for several years and on occasion, I would see a youth standing on the stairway, smoking a cigarette. I assumed that this dwelling was his home and he was not allowed to smoke indoors. When I retired, I began to walk more and observed that on a daily basis many young persons were going in and out of this home. I noted the address and checked on the Internet if this was a family home. I found out this was a shelter and temporary home for youth who are homeless.

Within a week of gaining this information, I phoned and asked if volunteers were needed to deliver any of the programs. I was invited for an interview and had the opportunity to inform the supervisor that I can assist young persons to develop employability skills such as building a strong resume, prepare for, and ace an interview, expand their network and know the labour market.

I know what it is like to loose one's job and also how difficult it is to obtain a job if you do not have the necessary skills. I envision that for homeless youth this is a major hurdle compounded by not having a permanent address. I wanted them to know that there is hope for their future, someone cares and I can be a part of the team helping them to move forward. I motivate them to believe in themselves even when no one seems to care, at a time in their lives when it is hard for them to even believe in themselves.

I gained accessed to this youth shelter as a volunteer to deliver education programs each Monday morning for four hours. I developed a curriculum where youth with different levels of education would have the ability to learn the skills required to access job opportunities. I wanted them to share their lived work experiences and build their knowledge from their learned experiences. The staff of the shelter and I agreed on ground rules to be in place during the education sessions. These rules were flexible so that the youth in attendance could add or change a few of the rules. For example a young person could go outside to have a cigarette only during the breaks but the group could decide the timing of the breaks. The setting was not called a classroom but a "knowledge center" where ideas are shared, discussions are respectful and each person takes away tools that will be useful in gaining employment.

A majority of these young persons did not complete high school so most discussions were around service employment, jobs in the trades and opportunities for increasing their education to venture out into the labour market. Some youth had been employed by family members, had therefore not developed a resume or participated in interviews. Others had been working at minimum wage jobs and the organizations downsized or the young person was unable to work regularly due to medical reasons. Some had not worked since dropping out of high school.

Topics of discussion focused on how unemployment could be a great challenge but also be an opportunity to gain new skills and move into new areas in the job market. Each group consisted of six young persons so that they could be encouraged to share confidentially and build trust within the group. The first hour of the discussion is spent on talking about self and what it means to be unemployed vs. being employed.

Some young people verbalized that it was hard to find employment because they lack the skills that are required for the job market they would like to enter. Some worry about missing relationships and friends. For example, unable to take a girlfriend to a movie or for dinner, others talk about being depressed and lonely.

We used the forum as opportunities to discuss how to overcome those barriers by accessing the hundreds of resources that the government provides for unemployed youth. Many were unaware of community resources and now learned how to access them. In this context, every participant had the opportunity to identify their skills and explore options to prepare for accessing the appropriate job market.

For those who had worked and lost their jobs due to medical reasons or organization downsizing, most of their focus was developing revised resumes and preparing to ace the interviews. They learn very quickly that their resume is the greatest marketing tool that connects them to employers. It is actually the face that that an employer sees and if they like what they see, there is a good chance for an interview. When building their resumes, I guide them in knowing that employers set timeframes for filling vacant positions and hundreds of applicants are vying for the same job opening. Their resumes need to stand out from others and include most of the job skills that the employer requires. They are encouraged to discuss who they are and what skills they are bringing to the company and to include some of these information in the their resumes. Employers are only interested in hiring individuals who bring benefits to their organizations, not liabilities.

The young persons then review and practice skills for a successful interview knowing that this is another great marketing tool that must be used to obtain employment. They learn the DOs and DON'Ts for successful interviews such as questions that employers are prohibited to ask related to age, gender, religion, country of origin and marital status. They also discuss attire to wear for the interview such as clean clothes that fit well and appropriate to the job for which they applied. Wearing blue jeans to be interviewed for a job in the office would not be appropriate, however this would be okay for a job interview to become a handy man. To enhance their engagement and ensure that they are learning I often ask "Can you imagine a forklift driver showing up for an interview at a construction site in a suite and tie and a business executive showing up at the bank in overalls and steel toe shoes?" These discussions usually emit much laughter and firm commitment for dressing appropriately.

They are also reminded that grooming and personal hygiene are also vital. The employer does not want to hire a dirty, smelly, unkempt individual. They are reminded that there is a need to project a good image. If not the employer may think that if the young person were unable to take care of self, would not be able to take care of the job.

In a relaxed and calm environment, they are supported in practicing all the skills they are taught. In the age of technology, it is amazing how many youth are homeless but do have their cell phones fully charged. Some make notes on their phones and all have access to computers at the shelter, to build their resumes.

Navigating the labour market in search of the right job can be very challenging but young persons are encouraged to use the 3 Ps to help them: Persistence, Positive and Polite. I am so pleased each week when I return to the shelter, I reunite with one or two of the young persons who had attended the education sessions. I receive a report back that he/ she has now developed a wining resume and would like me to review it or one may ask to practice some added interviewing skills. I know that I am making a difference and impacting lives of these young persons.

Living in a youth shelter though temporary, is one of the good decision a youth makes when that youth can no longer reside in a family home. It is much better than living on the streets where he could be robbed or beaten, abused or become involved in the drug trade or prostitution. Good things happen in the shelter. A few youth are reconnected with family supports during visits and though may not return home, they at least have someone to call in an emergency. Others are provided with counseling especially those with mental health challenges and low self- esteem.  Many gain work skills and are connected to housing. A shelter is often seen as a terrible place to be but this is where some young person starts life anew. All of us in society can help support vulnerable youth facing multiple barriers through mentoring, recreational and after school program. Some of us have the skills to support parents to increase parenting capacity. This world would be a better place' each one reach one'.

Advisory Board for Homeless Strategies in the Region:

"BEING HOMELESS IS DEFINED as a situation where one has no fixed address and is spending time in emergency shelters or places not meant for human habitation. This definition also includes individuals exiting institutions such as the child welfare system, mental health facilities, hospitals and correctional institutions. Being at imminent risk of homelessness is defined as a situation where one's current housing will end within two months; for whom no subsequent residence has been identified and is at immediate risk of moving into an emergency shelter or a place not meant for human habitation". (Region of Peel Target Population)

I live in the region that is often perceived as an area where rich folks live. This could not be further from the truth. Yes, there are some residents that are 'well off' but a large majority is middle class and many are homeless. In the major cities, it is easier to identify folks who are homeless, as they are not only sleeping on the sidewalks and remain there throughout the day. They frequent the food banks daily and many are occupying beds nightly in the shelters; most are visible. In my region, they are found sleeping in their cars, underneath bridges or coach surfing amongst friends and obtaining meals from food banks and other support services. Some work only minimum wage to take care of their families and is one paycheck away from becoming homeless. They are not always visible.

So why do I care about folks that are homeless? I was homeless twice as a teenager and know what it is like not to have a home that provides basic needs that are required to survive. I know that if loving and caring individuals did not help me to regain my self-esteem and to focus on my strengths I could not have done so alone. I wear my heart on my sleeves for folks who are homeless.

For individuals who work minimum wage, those who are experiencing mental illness, some from broken family units where there is domestic abuse, and those who struggle with alcohol and drug addictions, being homeless has become an intricate part of their lives. Most struggle with paying monthly rents and when they are evicted from their homes, the situation gets worse as they are unable to now find a first and last rent to re-enter. Homelessness can happen to anyone that is what Joan said when I listened to her story. She used to work and owned a four-bedroom house but she lost her home, thanks to gambling and family troubles. She continued that she went from riches to rags and found a temporary home in a woman's shelter.

As a passionate, and ardent community volunteer, I want to make a difference. I read an advertisement in the local newspaper where the homelessness partnering strategy advisory board was seeking a volunteer who would be willing to spend time assisting with support services and capital project funding reviews. I applied, submitted my resume and a short biography.  I was welcomed aboard to be an integral part of the team. Support services in the region are encouraged to submit proposals for projects that seek to prevent and reduce homelessness. These support services must demonstrate that they will be able to improve the self-sufficiency of homeless individuals and families and those at imminent risk of homelessness through individualized services.

I love being engaged in reading the proposals and sharing feedback with our team in making the decision for which organizations receive funding annually. Not only do I give back to my community but also I learn about the work that many organizations do to help folks that are homeless. I have added lots more knowledge to my toolbox about support services in my region. I can now be proactive by referring those who need the services before they become homeless and also those who homeless or at imminent risk of becoming homeless.


How Do Nursing Grads Obtain Employment Without Further Mentorship to Access the Job Market
I Fill the Gap:
When I graduated from nursing school many years ago, I was blessed to have a full time job waiting for me at the hospital

where I previously worked and that was instrumental in helping me to become an RN. I did not present a resume nor did I have an interview to gain employment.

Many new grads are exiting universities with very high levels of education but are not taught how to develop the tools that will open up job opportunities for them.

I am a member of the Registered Nurses Association of Ontario, Peel Chapter. Our vision is that "we speak out for nursing and speak out for health". I have chosen to equip as many new grads as possible with the skills they require to access the job market in a timely manner. I recently read an email from one of my nursing colleague, Karen, who wrote " Norma I know that you are so busy but I really need your help with a new grad. She has developed a resume that I think will not have any employer offering her an interview. She has outlined all her clinical placements to prove to the potential employer that she has the skills but I think she needs more than. I have told her that you have helped many new grads gain these skills. You have even assisted me to update my own resume for this new job that I am enjoying. Would you have any time to connect with her and help with developing a good resume and how to manage an interview? I would love to share your contact, do write back soon".

How could I ever say no to such a request! It is such a delight to see folks reach their potential. I have read several resumes that were developed by nursing graduates where they have outlined every new skill they learned, but failed to state their accomplishments and also to recognize that some of the skills they gained were basic and can be delivered by a personal support worker or a registered practical nurse. The employer is looking for an RN who will lead and build a multidisciplinary team, participate in and enhance the development of a variety of students, one who has demonstrated leadership skills in collaborating with clients and their families toward good health outcomes.

I have met with new graduates in their homes, my home office, church basements, many coffee outlets and restaurants, to assist them in developing expertise to access the jobs market. I have received many thank you cards and letters as these nurses have gained employment in their chosen areas of health care. Some have moved away from the province to gain employment in areas across Canada. I encourage nurses to go to the areas most in need and do not necessarily stay in the city unless they have an established family unit who would be unable to move. What makes me most proud is when a nurse who I have mentored and coached begins to mentor and coach others for success.

Crystal writes in a letter, "Norma, you are so kind and caring. You helped me to see my strengths, when I thought only of my weaknesses. I had gone to four interviews and no employer offered me a job. I am working as an aide in a long-term care home and felt so sad that I was unable to use my registered nurse's skills. A light bulb went off when you showed me that my resume did not portray me as a registered nurse but as an aide. Thank you so much, I am excited that at last I have an interview in a week towards obtaining a job in my preferred field. Do continue to help others fulfill their dreams".

I know that I am making a difference in this volunteer role because I am seeing great outcomes. I received two resumes this past week, a day apart, sent for my review. I take four hours to review and rewrite each resume. I then connect with the new grad nurse and obtain permission to revamp their resumes. These two nurses I have planned to meet with them to explain the changes to their resumes and coach them in preparing and managing interviews. Most of my nursing colleagues know that I do this volunteer work and will continue to be my referral sources.

### Centre for Young Parents

THIS CHARITABLE ORGANIZATION in a variety of ways provides support, education and counseling for single families. The clients are between the ages of 15 – 30 years, pregnant or parenting mothers, fathers and caregivers for children 0 – 6 years of age. All services offered are free. As a volunteer, I actively participate in the GAP program (Grow as Parents). I educate participants on how they can become successful parents. We discuss situations, which are happening at home such as the challenge of toilet training.  Some parents are learning the approaches while others see themselves as 'trying and failing' especially when neighbours ask, "when are you going to potty train Joseph?"

I am an ardent admirer of the advice given by Barbara Coloroso in her book titled "Kids are Worth It". I use the approaches outlined in this wonderful book to support parents to learn how to potty train their toddlers. I share stories of the 'brick-wall approach' where parents want to take complete control of the process of toilet training even before the child is physically ready. The parent may place the child on the potty every ten minutes throughout the day and offer rewards when the child goes. However if there are any accidents, the parent becomes frustrated and may punish for making mistakes. I stress that this approach is the wrong way to toilet train a child. The parents are encouraged to see their own children as special and strive not to compare them with others that are of the same age. For example they are encouraged to refrain from saying things such as "big girls don't pee in their pants; John does not wet his pants anymore, why can't you" A brick-wall parent set up battles and the child can choose to please or resist.

I engage parents in discussion around the 3 Ps of toilet training that are, prepare, practice and patience. Prepare; both parents and child need to be ready to take on the task of toilet training. Parents are to be ready to help their child because he/ she is ready to be helped. The parents then ask me, how do I know when they are ready? My response, most children are physically ready between the ages of eighteen months and two and a half years. Some children may be late as three and a half years – four years old. The basic signs of being physically ready is when your child is able to stay dry for long periods throughout the day and bowel movements are fairly regular.

Our discussion then moves into willingness of the child to be toilet trained. A child may reach these milestones when training could be started but may not be ready. A good sign of willingness is when the child asks to have the diaper changed immediately after urinating or having a bowel movement. Next is the child's ability to communicate when he or she needs to go. The child may say, mom I need to go potty now! I inform these young parents that what I am sharing are guidelines of when potty training can occur, as each child is unique, however when these three things come together, potty training is much easier.

Parents have other questions such as when a potty- chair should be used or a potty -seat placed on the toilet. Most often it is easier to start training by encouraging your child to use a potty- chair. Parents can even placed a teddy to sit on the potty when demonstrating how the child should sit. We also discuss easily managed outfit for a child such as cotton training pants that can be pulled up and down by the child. Parents are encouraged to have on hand lots of toilet paper. Parents are encouraged to assist with hygiene when the child is learning to use the potty. As they grow older, they usually feel comfortable taking over that role.  For some unknown reason, kids do learn to use toilet paper well as they will also practice wiping their stuffed toys. Washing of hands after bathroom use is very important so a handy safe step stool to allow little Jean to reach the sink to wash hands with soap and water. That same step stool can be used later when Jean advances to using the potty seat on the toilet, it can be used for resting her feet.  I remind parents often that there is no one right way to potty train. Find what is best for parent and child. The key to remember is that as a parent you are helping your child take control of his/her body. Your child just needs your help, guidance and support.

During the education session, participants are involved in discussions and props are used to demonstrate some of the techniques. The infants and toddlers are often enjoying recreation activities with other volunteers so that parents can focus on learning. Surprisingly during these sessions, a toddler walks into the classroom and says out loud "Mommy I have to go potty". Once each month I am a volunteer 'potty trainer'. Young families especially those who are first time parents do appreciate this support. Their smiles tell me that they have gained added tools for taking care of their children.

## Supporting Families who are Experiencing Alzhemier's Disease

ALZHEIMER'S IS THE MOST common form of dementia, a general term for memory loss and other intellectual abilities serious enough to interfere with activities of daily life. This disease accounts for 60 – 80 percent of dementia cases. As our population age all over the world, we are finding that folks are living longer and many are showing signs and symptoms of this disease. Nursing homes are filled; so many families try their best to provide care at home for anyone who is affected with this disease.

Families need additional help when the individual who is affected is demonstrating behaviours that cannot be managed without someone providing 24- hour care in the home.

Alzheimer's disease is not a normal part of aging although the greatest known risk factor is increasing age. This disease worsens over time, is progressive and the symptoms gradually worsen over a number of years. In the early stages, memory loss is mild but with late-stage Alzheimer's, individuals loose the ability to carry on a conversation and respond appropriately to their immediate environment. There are no simple solutions for caring for someone with any kind of dementia. Each person presents a different challenge each day as they experience memory loss. There is no cure for the disease but there are many ways to provide loving care, which promotes the dignity and self-esteem of the individual.

Maya Angelou says, " Life is pure adventure and the sooner we realize that, the quicker we will be able to treat life as an art: to bring all our energies to each encounter, to remain flexible enough to notice and admit when what we expected to happen did not happen. We need to remember that we can invent new scenarios as frequently as they are needed". Caregivers and families of individuals who are affected by Alzheimer's disease must be creative to promote good quality of life for them especially knowing no one expects to encounter this disease and those who have are missing their short term memories but have some intact long term memories.

EXAMPLE

Mary is 86 years old and lives in a long- term care home. She has been diagnosed with Alzheimer's disease for four years.

This morning after she had her breakfast, she hurries to get her handbag. When asked, where are you going Mary? She responds, I am going to work. A care provider who do not understand that Mary is using her long term memory of having to get her handbag before heading out to work, would respond incorrectly to Mary. The response may be, you no longer go to work, and you are living in a long- term care home. Mary then becomes very upset and restates that she is ready for work. The best response where Mary and her situation are validated is by attempting every means of clue gathering, puzzle piecing and improvisation to assist her. There is a responsibility to assist Mary to re-experience herself. It is good to recognize and be familiar with the person's life history and the reality the person might be living an any given moment. The response could be simply; Mary, I know that you need your handbag when you are going to work (validating), lets have a seat over here and tell me about your work, what did you do at your workplace (helping to relive past experiences). Mary is now allowed to retrieve memories and feelings that will assist her cope with the situation at hand. Often times after the discussion, Mary will not remember that she wanted to go to work. Remembering that it is our reality that Mary cannot go to work, it is not her reality. Mary returns her handbag to her room and participates in recreational activities.

I am a past president of the Alzheimer's society in my region and gained an incredible amount of knowledge when I was in that volunteer role. I now use my knowledge at least twice weekly to assist families to connect with community resources or to learn safe ways of supporting their families at home.

My cell phone rings and I check to see who is sending me a text. It is one of my best friends who has recently returned from vacation. Perhaps she wants to share some of the great events that occurred while she was away but the text says " can you call me as soon as possible or where can I call you now"? The urgency of the text message had me scrambling to the land phone. I called my friend Dorothy and she says, I need help with my mom. I know you have given me some advice before but nothing I do today is working. When asked, tell me what your mom is doing today, she responded, I have not been able to get her to eat, she keeps crying for her dad to come home. What can I do? When asked how she has been responding to her mom, she reports that she said, your dad is coming home later.

We then discussed why the word 'later' has no meaning for her mom since her disease is advancing and she cannot relate to time aligned with events. I asked if her mom was dressed warmly to go for a walk. She said yes. I advised her to ask her mom to go with her to the restaurant. When I assisted my friend to develop strategies to keep her mom at home as long as she is able, she shared that mom loved going to a small restaurant in the neighbourhood for meals. I now suggest that she takes her mom to the restaurant that is within walking distance of their home. Her mom could get some exercise and also may eat a meal at the restaurant since it is small facility and often quiet. She thanked me and took her mom to the restaurant. This approach worked out very well, her mom enjoyed the walk and as Dorothy reported back, she had the largest meal in a long time. We are reminded daily that what works with one individual may never work with another. Also what works one day may not work the next with the same individual.

I have a coffee meeting with my friend soon to help her to do some planning for her mom's ongoing health care. I could hear the panic in her voice when she had tried and was unable to support her mom through a small crisis. I worry that she may not be able to manage larger issues such as wandering, aggressive behaviours and severe confusion. We have invited her brother to join us for this conversation. He does not want his mom to enter a nursing home. A decision has to be made to obtain more support for Dorothy, so that as the care giver she does not get burnt out and become ill herself. I am hoping that the outcome of this planned discussion will be a decision making time for added in home support or to consider completing the necessary application forms for entry into a nursing home.

In this volunteer role, I also support families who would like to have the individual with Alzheimer's stay at home but they need a vacation. In the Region of Peel there is a very a very dedicated and caring Alzheimer's society that in collaboration with stakeholders, developed and manages a 24 hour-vacation home for individuals having dementia and whose care givers need to take a break. Taking a break from caring

often called respite or respite care is important for anyone providing day-to-day care for someone with this disease. It can
be physically and emotionally tiring and stressful. Families
and caregivers can easily become isolated from social contacts,
particularly if they are unable to have a rest, go out, attend
to business or go on a holiday. This vacation home provides
a much-needed break from the responsibilities and demands
of caring for someone with dementia. Many people find that
a regular break means they can recharge and avoid burn out,
and it may delay placement in a long- term care home. A family member commented that not only did this respite home
provided overnight respite for a block of days, but it also made
it possible for her to carry out career-related activities and responsibilities that required travel out of the country.

Rosemary Dunn says, a lifetime of experience and skill
is a foundation of one's self-esteem. This must be preserved
and encouraged when so much else is lost. Families greatly
appreciate supports that they receive from volunteers to care
for family members.

## Helping Children with Challenging Behaviours Reach Their Potential

> *If you expect the worst, you'll get the worse, and*
> *if you expect the best, you'll get the best"*

> Norman Vincent Peale.

YOUNG LIVES ON THE LINE: You can make a difference is the title of my first book in which I explored why certain challenging behaviours occur in our adolescents. I use these researched findings to assist families to support and love their teens.  Knowing the root causes of behaviours in this age group, I am able to examine why similar behaviours occur in younger children and work with parents to develop strategies to manage the behaviours.

> Barbara Kaiser and Judy Sklar, defines challenging behaviours "as any behaviour that interferes with a child's cognitive, social or emotional development, is harmful for a child, his peers or adults and places a child at high risk for later social problems or school failure".

I am not sure why parents and especially grand parents of single mothers seek me out for support. I am so very humbled that they do this, most often from hearing what others say about the ways in which I have assisted them.  Reflecting on my childhood, where I received no guidance around having good behaviour, I am so happy that no one perceived me to have had any challenging behaviours. I believe that behaviors that are aggressive, antisocial or disruptive greatly impact the child and anyone who comes into contact with that child. These kinds of behaviours place children in danger by preventing them from learning what they need to know to succeed in school and get along with others. Some parents and the teachers in the schools find themselves at loss, unable to figure out how to turn things around, how to   make the situation tenable while helping the child to get back on track and behaving appropriately.   Even if a mother is most confident and experienced in managing her child's behaviours, there are times when there are doubts on how to deal with some of these kinds of behaviours. I provide education sessions in the middle school and meet with parents over coffee or talk with them on the phone about managing children's challenging behaviours. I remind parents and teachers that this kind of behaviour serves the child well. For example, because a mother is embarrassed at her child's behaviour, it may prompt her to purchase a chocolate bar for the child who screams and has a lengthy tantrum in the supermarket because he had been refused the chocolate when he first asked to have one. As this child receives a reward for this negative behaviour, the child learns to use this behaviour more and becomes skillful over time; it may become more difficult to change.

However a child who demonstrates ongoing challenging behaviour does have real needs and these have to be addressed and managed before the child can succeed. As a parent, you usually know if your child is able and willing to perform a task, that child will need little supervision or support from you. When the child is able but unwilling to perform the task, then this child may have the skills and knowledge but lack the motivation to do what you asked. You will find ways to shore up the child's willingness and bolster his confidence. The real challenge occurs when behaviour occurs over and over and as a parent you struggle with the right response, this impedes your ability to focus on the underlying cause of the behaviour and you want to address and manage what you are presented; in fact you become ineffective. In so many schools and homes, kids with social, emotional and other behavioral challenges are still poorly understood and treated in ways that sometimes makes the situation worse.

## An Example of Managing Challenging Behaviour:

I WAS AT THE HAIRDRESSERS and while she was styling my hair, she looked at the book that I was reading and asked, is that a book that can help my seven year old and me? I responded, it depends on what kind of help you both need. She informs me that her seven year old is a tyrant and will not do what she tells him nor does he listen to his teacher. He throws his toys, he runs around the classroom and when he is at home, she is unable to get him to sit for a meal nor do his homework. I paused, and said; tell me again, your seven year old is a tyrant? She said yes he is! I informed her that I have frequent discussions with teachers and parents to assist them in supporting their children through challenging behaviours. I asked if she would like my help and she said a resound YES I would! I exchanged contact information with her, asked her to connect with me when she was on her day off and to grant me one favor for that day. She responded; I am listening. I asked her to immediately stop calling her son a tyrant and to look at him as a loving seven-year and always use his name when speaking to him and eliminate the word tyrant from her vocabulary. I then learned that her son's name is Jason.

I received an email that same afternoon from my hairdresser and she asked if we could meet the following day for coffee near her workplace. We talked for a while on the phone to ensure that she would be willing to share confidentially the challenging behaviours that are presented by Jason and she would hone some of the suggestions and strategies I would provide to support her son in eliminating or at least decreasing the challenging behaviours. We met for coffee and I learned more about Jason. He is a very handsome caring child, loves his mom and is not involved with his father. He has no sibling and seeks his mom's attention at all times. She sees this as being irritating and an attention seeker. At school he screams and hit other children in his class. When the teacher sends him to the office he gets more upset and says he hates the teacher. He refuses to go to school most days and says his teacher does not like him. She punishes him when he does not sit quietly at the table, he is sent to his room.

I informed my new friend that Jason will do well if he can; he seems to be lacking some thinking skills and not those skills that are involved in traditional reading, writing and math. He seems to be lacking the cognitive skills which allows him to regulate his emotion, understand how his behaviour such as hitting, impacts his classmates and he does not have the words to let anyone know something is wrong. Jason may have a developmental delay or a learning disability.

She would need help from a social worker or a school psychologist to help develop strategies and work closely with her and Jason to implement and monitor outcomes. I asked her to spend as much time as possible showing love to her son, try to understand some of his behaviour, seek to help him to use words to describe what is happening and do not call him a tyrant. She promised to connect with the school to make an appointment and have a discussion with the school team so that she could gain support to help both Jason and herself.

I am hoping for a good outcome for Jason and for his mother and I am happy to have the opportunity to assist another mother and child. I am convinced that most children do their best when they can. The vast majority of kids with challenging behaviours already want to behave the right way. They do not need to be punished, suspended or deprived of their education. They are having difficulty mastering the skills required for becoming effective in handling life's social, emotional and behavioural challenges. I know for sure that in every challenging experience there is an opportunity to learn and grow.

I love what our Office of the Provincial Advocate for Children and Youth does to positively impact the lives of youth and their families. I have included a small portion of their 2016 annual report to the provincial legislature about youth in care of the Children's Aid Societies:

## What They Heard from Young People

If you ask young people what's going on in their lives and how it could be better, they have plenty to say…and their opinions and views are as individual as their circumstances. Still, we know that young people's concerns often revolve around core sources of conflict or pain. For example, they are not allowed to see their files; they may be denied access to their biological parents without knowing why; they may be moved from one group home to the next with no explanation; they are unaware of their rights; some feel unsafe where they live, or have been abused or mistreated; and because of their disconnection from close family and frequent transfers, many feel isolated and lost. As they grow up and face transitions from care to independence, many tell us they feel unprepared for the challenges ahead.

Situations like these cause young people to get into trouble with the law. Many who are incarcerated came to jail through the Children's Aid Society pipeline.

## What I Heard from Registered Nurses
From an RN community member:

Norma, when I came to audit your infection control at the youth-custody center, I met you as the manager of the medical unit for youth. I was struck by your compassion and deep understanding of who these young people were, and why they'd ended up incarcerated. While you were telling me about the reality of their daily lives and what you all were trying to do for them, I remember wondering how you had the strength and courage every day to face, not the youth, but the administration who were obviously in such a different headspace than you were. You saw the youth as individuals who had the opportunity for change and growth; young people who had been disadvantaged since birth, who needed support, structure, education, and love. Your administration saw them as problems to be dealt with, and demonstrated underlying judgment and prejudice. Speaking with you and seeing your obvious passion and commitment inspired me to follow my passion more fully. Shortly after our meeting, I applied and went in to a new role as an RN. You reminded me that the art of nursing was equally as important as the science at a critical time.

From an RN staff member:

You are one of the most inspiring, positive people I have met in my life. The impact you have had on me to rekindle my hope and optimism—that things will work out if you have faith, are kind to people, and follow your instinct. This is something I thought I had lost a little while when I first met you, and every time we see each other, it is like a breath of fresh air. Thank you, Norma, for the person you are.

## What I Heard from Physicians
From a physician:

I am so happy to see that you're writing another book, one that is dedicated to your impactful career as a nurse. I love the title! As a physician I can appreciate the need for sensible shoes, and how they can make traveling from one place more efficient. I think sensible shoes are a reference to your courageous and sensible nature.

From another physician:

I think what stood out for me, Norma, was your genuine care and concern for the rehabilitation of the youth, even when it seemed that the administration was moving away from rehab and moving to jail-like structure. You kept fighting for the youth until the day you retired. You were trying to rehabilitate them, to get them back to being active members of society, more than they were interested (in doing). They will thank you in the future when they realize it also. The fact you hired me to go on that journey with you is a special thing for me also.

# Lifelong Learning

*You are truly an amazing person and a great
ambassador for our region! The only wish I have
in my life is to have an impact like you and to
leave this world a better place than when I came.
Congratulations on your accomplishments.*

—Senior Police Officer

As a nursing student, there were not adequate hours
during the three years of training to learn about every aspect
of therapeutic relationship, medical diagnosis, and clinical
practice required for each patient. As a nurse, I am committed
to lifelong learning. Each day technology, research, and
evidence-based practices bring about new ways to enhance
the health care of our citizens. I change some of my practice
approaches to ensure that the nursing care I provide is holistic and meets the needs of individual patients.

I had the opportunity to attend school at the age of eight, and that was when I learned to read. Prior to age eight, I lived with my grandmother on a farm and worked in the fields daily. Learning to read has instilled in me a love for gaining knowledge. I gained control of my world, and this gets better every day because of my ongoing learning and sharing acquired skills with every sector in my community.

There are many opportunities to gain further education, as this is a requirement for professional practice. Given that some educational forums are costly, and organizational budgets have decreased funding for ongoing education, I search for free or inexpensive workshops. I ensure the information gained enhances my knowledge to deliver effective health care. If funding is not available, I often ask about volunteer opportunities to assist the learners, and in that way I attend and participate.

As my knowledge increases, I acquire the skills to give exceptional care and become more engaged in ensuring that the best health care is given to our changing demographics.

Wisdom from one of my favorite authors, Jeff Keller:

The longer I live, the more I realize the impact of attitude on life. Attitude, to me, is more important than facts. It is more important than the past, than education, than money, than circumstances, than failures, than successes, than what other people think or say or do. It is more important than appearance, giftedness or skills. It will make or break a company…a church…a home.

The remarkable thing is we have a choice every day regarding the attitude we will embrace for that day. We cannot change our past…we cannot change the fact that people will act in a certain way. We cannot change the inevitable. The only thing we can do is play on the one string we have and that is our attitude.

I am convinced that life is 10 percent what happens to me and 90 percent how I react to it. And so it is with you…we are in charge of our ATTITUDES.

⸺∽⸺

## Plaques

- Alzheimer Society of Peel: Years of dedicated service and enhanced role of president of the society.
- Absolutely Fabulous Women of Peel: Excellence in community service.
- Jamaican Canadian Association of Nurses: Award of excellence, outstanding leadership in nursing.
- Ontario Black History Society, Rose Fortune Award: Dedicating a lifetime to helping at-risk youth rise up and live fulfilling lives.
- The Roy McMurtry Youth Center: In recognition and appreciation for years of service to at-risk youth.

## CERTIFICATES

- Completion from Volunteer Training Center: Measuring success: how to evaluate the impact of volunteer engagement.
- Rockhurst University Continuing Education Center: Leadership and supervisory skills for women.
- Joseph Rotman School of Management, University of Toronto: Leadership development.
- Centennial College: Forensic Nursing.
- Participation, Crime Prevention Workshop: Safe City Mississauga, focus on youth.
- York University, Osgoode Hall Law School: Healthcare law.
- Participation: Twenty-first psychogeriatric team exchange.
- Sheridan College: Managing wandering behaviors in dementia.
- Successful Participation: Working successfully with toddlers in a volunteer role.
- Seventh-Day Adventist Church Recognition: Educating women on the management of behaviors in their teenagers.
- Sheridan College: Fundamentals of teaching and learning: network for innovation and leadership in education.
- Ontario Management Development Program: Leadership skills: focus on community outreach.

- Crime Prevention Police Academy Achievement: Focus on home and community safety.
- Achievement: Recognition for volunteering time and effort as a Passages speaker in Canada.
- Graduation: Completed course in mental-health first aid: demonstrated ability to initiate help to people experiencing mental-health problems.
- Elder Abuse Protocol Training Completion: Identify, prevent, and educate about abuse.
- Recognition: Volunteered as a medic at the Toronto 2015 Pan Am/Parapan Am Games.
- Heritage Mississauga Awards: Contributions and achievements in the preservation of our community heritage.

## OTHER RECOGNITIONS

- Registered Nurses' Association of Ontario: Distinction of quarter-century club member for loyalty and support over the past twenty-five years.
- Registered Nurses' Association, Peel Chapter: Lifetime achievement award for outstanding work in health care.
- Registered Nurses' Association of Ontario: Leadership award in nursing administration: "Leading a diverse team of nursing leaders to positively impact patient care. Ensured an effective clinical work

environment and all aspects of care include best practices."

* Registered Nurses' Association: HUB Fellowship for demonstrating leadership potential and a commitment to the nursing profession: "She proactively develops relationships with local newspaper reporters and Members of Provincial Parliament to ensure the public and decision makers are aware of the role of nurses and their importance in the healthcare system."

* Toronto Star Nightingale Awards: Nominated five consecutive years by staff, past patients and their families, and nursing colleagues from all levels of health-care organizations: "You have touched the lives of others by ensuring the highest standards of professional care and by going that extra step for families and your community."

* Member of Parliament of the Ontario Legislature: "On behalf of the valuable contribution you and your colleagues of the Registered Nurses' Chapter of Peel have made to the Ontario healthcare system, your tireless dedication and unwavering commitment to the health and safety of all Ontarians sets you apart from other professionals."

* Member of Provincial Parliament of the Ontario Legislature: Leading women building communities: "The province of Ontario proudly recognizes you for your exceptional community leadership to improve the lives of girls and women in Ontario."

NORMA NICHOLSON IS A PUBLISHED author, speaker, educator, community advocate, and youth and adult mental-health
expert. She is a registered nurse with a BA in sociology and
psychology from the University of Toronto and an MA in
adult education from Central Michigan University.

She has been a nursing leader for forty years in a variety
of health-care sectors. She is a lifelong learner and has ad-
vanced from a registered practical nurse to an outstanding
registered nurse leader with a postgraduate degree.

She has served on the boards of many large and impactful
organizations and has received many prestigious awards as a
volunteer for her community engagement.

Her first published book, *Young Lives on the Line: You
Can Make a Difference*, came out of her passion for making
a difference in the lives of marginalized and underserved
youth. She dedicates a minimum of fifteen hundred hours
annually to community activities.

68626627R00075